A Place Called Self

A Place Called Self

Women, Sobriety, and
Radical Transformation

Stephanie Brown, Ph.D.

with Yvonne Pearson

HAZELDEN

Hazelden
Center City, Minnesota 55012-0176

1-800-328-0094
1-651-213-4590 (Fax)
www.hazelden.org

Library of Congress Cataloging-in-Publication Data
Brown, Stephanie, 1944–
    A place called self : women, sobriety, and radical transforma-
tion / Stephanie Brown, with Yvonne Pearson.
        p. cm.
    ISBN - 13: 978-1-59285-098-3

    1. Recovering alcoholics—Psychology. 2. Women alcoholics—
Psychology. 3. Alcoholics—Rehabilitation. I. Pearson, Yvonne.
II. Title.

HV5275.B76 2004
616.86'103—dc22

                                                    2004047346

All vignettes found in this book were created by the author to represent
common experiences of women in recovery from alcoholism or other drug
addiction. Any resemblance to specific persons, living or dead, or specific
events is coincidental.

08 07   6 5 4 3

Cover design by Theresa Gedig
Interior design by Rachel Holscher
Typesetting by Stanton Publication Services, Inc.

For my mother,
and in memory of my father,
with love and compassion.

Contents

Acknowledgments

I have said thank you many times over many years, and now I have the opportunity to do so again. Immediately, a great swell of gratitude leaps up in me as I think about the process of writing this book and the extraordinary gifts I received in working with two incredible editors. Rebecca Post of Hazelden suggested this project and helped me craft an outline and a style that would speak to women everywhere. Yvonne Pearson, an exquisite writer, worked step-by-step with me to make it a reality. Both of these partnerships were challenging, invigorating, and always touching as I learned to speak to readers in a less academic, more personal voice.

I carry ages-old gratitude to all the supporters I have had personally and professionally for more than thirty years as I found my own way in recovery and, in a parallel and interwoven way, began thinking and writing theoretically about what recovery is. In a sense, my own journey is reflected in this book.

Some of these longtime supporters require repeated mention now, as I think about gratitude. At the top of the list are countless individuals in AA, Al-Anon, and many other Twelve Step programs who have shared their "experience, strength, and hope" with me over the years as research subjects, clients, and friends. I have been blessed to see recovery up close and to know people who have been on this road for many, many years.

I have also been blessed to work professionally with therapists and other helping professionals, seeking to bridge what used to be a cavernous gap between addiction knowledge and traditional mental health treatments. Today, there is much more collaboration and understanding across these disciplines. Many more therapists have now seen long-term recovery up close too, and the impact has been extremely positive. I'm so grateful to my colleagues who worked closely with me in my early days at Stanford, and to those who have been with me over the last fifteen years at the Addictions Institute, for their commitment to work with people in recovery and to carry a new message to professionals.

Finally, in the naming, I must include the National Association for Children of Alcoholics. I was so lucky to be part of this founding group, and I have been lucky to see this grassroots movement grow into a solid, strong voice for all children and adult children affected by a parent's alcoholism.

To all the others I haven't named or renamed, I say thank you again. I feel a deep gratitude to everyone for the life I've been given. And to those who share it with me, I offer a final special mention. As always, thanks to my husband, Robert Harris, and our daughter, Makenzie, for their love, humor, and understanding.

Stephanie Brown

Prologue

I was born in the middle of my life. It was March 19, 1971. I was twenty-six years old. The previous night, March 18, I had what was to be my last drink. I did not know it at the time, nor did I know it the next day. Over several weeks, then months and years, this pair of average and insignificant days would come to clearly mark the most important turning point in my life.

I am one of those individuals who was *reborn*, a word I never trusted. But that is what happened. And so I join the ranks of the second-comers, the transformed and converted, whether I like it or not. I have come to like it.

The story of my life, so far, is two stories, like night and day in many ways, but tied forever by the liquid umbilical cord of alcohol. It was drinking—beginning at age sixteen with a glass of wedding champagne—that gave me life, and it was drinking that ended it, ten years later. Until that magic first glass, I lived in a swamp of other people's drinking. My childhood was completely dominated by my parents' alcoholism and the confused, terrifying, humiliating world that was my family. I felt like an orphan in an underground, drunken fog. After my first drink, the fog lifted. I found my family, I found my roots, and I was home.

The worst years of my life—the drinking years—were also the best. Closeness, affection, and a sense of belonging were mine. For, despite the horrors, this was a loving home.

My separation from alcohol on that windy Friday afternoon in March also marked inevitably and completely my separation from my family, and the beginning step-by-step, starting-from-scratch process of growing up again. On the twenty-first anniversary of my abstinence, I planted a rose bush in my honor and in memory of my father. It was a bittersweet "coming of age" tribute. There was no one from my first family to share in this passage. My second family, my husband and daughter, mark each anniversary with me. As observers, they are wonderfully dutiful in acknowledging this day. But they weren't there during my first life, and they did not live it with me. They have only the "after" picture, which they like a lot. They can't imagine me drunk. Thank God.

I can. I remember it well. But, within my first family, I remembered it alone. When I stopped drinking and declared myself an alcoholic, I severed the cord—the most important bond to my family. If I were to be an alcoholic, I would be one alone.

In 1965, I was in New York on my first twenty-first birthday. Lonely and homesick, I celebrated by myself, rhythmically pouring my habitual cocktail with an added silent toast to mark this day. But it was nothing, not even a real passage in this state where adulthood began at eighteen. The grocer in the corner deli rang up my usual pint and that was it. How could I tell him that I had just turned twenty-one? And so I felt alone on my second twenty-first birthday, this time separated from my first family by the gulf in our realities. As I have known deeply over all these years, I orphaned myself on that day in March 1971. I gave up the only link to comfort and love that I had ever known. But I also got my life.

These first pages ring full of such sorrow that I want to go back and say "no." I want to say "it wasn't so bad" as I have carefully maintained all these years. But actually, it was. It is only in the last few years that I have been able to tolerate looking backward to unravel the pain. Through the early years of abstinence, I maintained a romanticized view of my family, seeing the alcoholism as a tragic flaw that marred an otherwise ideal home. I was unable to see the dark side, and the filtered light of nostalgia only awakened in me a deep sense of loss and longings to go back home. But there was no remedy for this homesickness, and nostalgia was not something I dared risk. This undertow would pull me down.

In my early sobriety I constructed a history of facts called a drunkalogue. As an observer of my own life, I compiled that history quickly and accurately, for the first time acknowledging the realities of my own drinking and the alcoholic world in which I'd grown up. But this was a two-dimensional history, with any nostalgia carefully disguised. When I told my "story" in the infancy of my sobriety, I always cried. These were tears of relief. It would be many years before I would add tears of open grief, loss, and longing.

In the early days, I unhitched my story from feeling and, strangely, I unhitched it from my own experience and memory. I recalled drinking but not the feeling of being drunk. I recognized the painful craving for alcohol but could not openly long for the closeness that went with drinking.

Some years ago, talking with recovering friends, I said that I had never known guilt and sorrow before I started drinking and certainly not while I was drinking, which is pretty unusual. Bottomless guilt and sorrow are part of the wreckage of a drinking life.

Not mine. My guilt and sorrow began on the day I put down the glass, stared at the bottle, and knew for the very first time that I was an alcoholic. At that moment, one life ended and another began.

There was absolutely nothing special about Friday, March 19, as far as I know. I was not even waiting out a St. Patrick's Day hangover because I never celebrated this salute to alcohol. For over a year I had been questioning my drinking, worried that I might have a "problem." Panic attacks provided the terrifying experience of impending disaster and a physical sense of the ground crumbling beneath me. My world seemed to be coming to an end, though I could not see what death was in store for me.

During that year of questioning, I held on to the outstretched hand of therapy, with the hope that seeing clearly would restore my balance, relieve my anxiety, and bring me back to normal. It was not to be. I would never go back to that normal. Seeing clearly would keep me unbalanced for many years as I dug myself out of the grave of my family's alcoholism, a legacy and a birthright that had become my own.

Much of the time I lived in that underground, drunken fog, a real world I had watched growing up and joined so readily at age sixteen. It was a world of confusion, a world run by impulse and desperate primitive need, an often grotesque world held together by the logic of dreams. Reality could not be known and did not exist. Daylight merged with the dark of sleep, bringing confusion, condensation, and confabulation aboveground, the bricks and mortar of my family's life. It was a world of images, of smells and sounds, a world before words, replayed continuously, going nowhere.

As the early days of March 1971 unfolded, I sunk into a holding pattern of despair. Still, I did not know what was wrong. On Friday, the 12th, I matter-of-factly described to my therapist the inevitable, automatic steps of getting drunk that I would enact the next night. This was not an event I was looking forward to, nor one that gave me pleasure. It was a repeated descent into hell, a visit home I made all the time.

My therapist listened and said quite mildly that it sounded as if I saw no alternative, that I had no choice about drinking. Curious, but not particularly surprised, I agreed.

On Saturday night I proceeded to get drunk exactly as I had described it to my therapist, never considering any other possibility. Though I was sitting at a bar with friends, I felt completely alone and utterly hopeless. I had just watched myself get drunk. It wasn't the first time I had tuned in to observe this spectacle, but it was the first time I recognized my helplessness.

Over the next few days, I went on about my business, drinking my nightly cocktails with little ceremony and not much fun. I was about to say good-bye to my life's companion and to my entire family. But I did not know it yet.

Thursday night, March 18, found me in the Formica-tabled House of Yee, a Chinese diner. I had never eaten there before and would never return. I sat with the newspaper, the three-choice special, wooden chopsticks, and a bottle of beer. I rarely drank beer and didn't particularly like it, but it was the only alcohol available. As I ordered it, I thought to myself how well beer goes with chow mein.

I can't recall if I had a second beer. Seems like I did. That was all and I headed home.

On Friday, I was sick, sure I had the flu. Actually, I never knew if I really had the flu or not because I was almost always hungover. Drinking every day makes you sick.

I stayed in bed all day. At 5:00 P.M., the start of my usual cocktail hour, I got up and headed for the kitchen. It never occurred to me not to drink if I was sick. It was time to drink, and so I would.

I poured a glass of sherry, a suitable accompaniment to the flu, I thought, and raised my hand, lifting the glass to my lips. Halfway up, I paused, and heard my own quiet, certain voice: "You are doing this to yourself. No one else is responsible. You will drink yourself to death."

It was over. I put the glass down, and then the bottle. There would be no more from that day till this one, almost twenty-two years later.

That day was March 19, a day I mark with gratitude and awe every year, but rarely celebration. Though I got my life, I lost my family and I lost my childhood. I turned off the switch on a past that was completely soaked in alcohol, and I stayed away from home emotionally for many years. I turned the switch off on longing and the yellowed newsprint of nostalgia.

On a clear fall day seven months later, I woke up, calmly packed all of my belongings into my powder blue 1963 VW Bug, and drove away from my alcoholic husband and our alcohol-soaked marriage. I had never considered leaving until that morning.

A few weeks later, newly settled in a cheap, furnished apartment, looking out on Highway 101, I got a wake-up call that my father had died. Cardiac arrest. Alcoholism, I knew. And perhaps a broken heart, caused by me, I was sure. To this day, I do not know whether he died feeling abandoned by me or secure in the knowledge that I had gotten out.

A few days before he died, he had sat in my dark living room, worrying about the location and shabby furnishings. He would pay if I would move to a better area. "No thanks," I said, as if turning down a drink. I had never been so happy. Without alcohol for eight months, without an alcoholic mate for one month, on my own for the first time, I was starting over.

Stephanie Brown
March 1993

PART ONE

Welcome to Recovery

Chapter One

What Is Recovery?

When Anne went to her first Alcoholics Anonymous (AA) meeting, she repeated the familiar statement: "Hi. My name is Anne. I'm an alcoholic and I'm in recovery." She had quit drinking the day before, and so she dared to make the claim that she was in recovery. But was it true? Did quitting really mean that she was in recovery? Well yes, but only partially, because quitting is only a tiny piece of it. Recovery is so much more than quitting. Let's listen in on Anne twenty years later as she tells her story at a treatment center.

Recovery has held so many surprises for me. Some good. Some bad. I didn't know I could hurt so much. But I also didn't know I could love so much and be so loved. I had no idea recovery was also learning how to be in intimate relationships, learning how to have close, wonderful friends. Then there's my marriage. My husband and I have developed a rich life together. And—get this—I really like myself now. Learning about who I am and accepting me, that's been the hardest part of recovery—and the best. I wouldn't trade this path for anything in the world.

Recovery is a journey, a process, like the evolution of a wizened old tree, bent and blown and impossibly beautiful. You can see that the tree has suffered the ravages of time, and the ravages themselves have become part of its beauty. This is recovery.

Recovery is a radical change in the self, a transformation. It's a long and, yes, even painful process of developing a self that has been neglected and distorted over many years. Recovery may even be finding a self that has never been born.

For many women, their real selves are barely known, even to themselves, barely audible, barely visible, and woefully underdeveloped. If you are in recovery, you have a lot of work ahead of you, perhaps a lifetime's worth of work to catch up on. But wrapped in with the sweaty, grueling work of it is the joy you feel when you hear your own strong voice singing, unencumbered by shame or self-consciousness.

We will explore this long, painful, and joyous process in detail, but first, let's look at what, exactly, we mean when we say "women in recovery." Who are we talking about?

Who Is the Woman in Recovery?

In this book I'm talking about the woman who has been actively addicted to a substance, to a repeated compulsive behavior, or to an individual. If you are a woman who has stopped drinking, using other drugs, gambling, overeating, undereating, or behaving in a compulsive, out-of-control manner in a relationship, you are the woman I am talking about. You are a woman who has faced yourself and who has come to a realization that you have lost control and cannot regain it, if indeed you ever had control. You have come to accept the fundamental, deep reality that you are powerless over your own needs and your actions to meet those needs—your active addiction.

This book asks and answers one important question: What happens to the woman who stops her active addiction? This is the woman who has the challenging and perhaps frightening opportunity to start a transformational process of new growth and development called recovery.

Redefining Recovery

The dictionary defines *recovery* as a reclaiming or "return" of something lost. According to this definition, a woman recovering from addiction is reclaiming the health, sanity, and well-being that may have existed before she became addicted. But that's not quite right. Recovery is more like a starting over than a restoration of what was lost. This is because, for many women, the real self was never really developed. As she grows up, a woman in our world frequently becomes role-bound before she knows who she is. Like the "beauty" of a traditional Chinese woman's bound and stunted feet, the "beauty" demanded of a woman's personality requires that her self conforms to a shape that is not hers. So when she strips off the false self presented in her addiction, her real self is only partially there. She frequently finds instead a stunted person.

Recovery is a resumption of the work that was not completed when the woman was a girl. It is a coming into her own. It is an opportunity to resume the normal process of development that was sidetracked, perhaps first by constrained roles, perhaps by trauma, and then multiplied many times by hiding in the addiction. Her development was sidetracked by not accepting her needs as legitimate and not finding healthy ways to meet them, by not even knowing her needs. *And so this is what recovery is: a developmental process of finding and building a new self.* Recovery is a process of radical growth and change. When you are in recovery, you give birth to a new self. Is it any surprise, then, that it's painful and it takes time?

Myths of Recovery

Recovery involves a change in meaning of everything a woman knows. In recovery, you will transform the way you think about yourself as well as the way you think about life itself. Before we explore this further, let's talk about two of the traditional ways of thinking about recovery that are actually misleading: (1) recovery is moving from bad to good; and (2) dependence is bad and recovery means you are no longer dependent.

Bad to Good or False to Real?

Many women initially think that recovery means a move from bad to good. They think that being addicted is evidence of shameful neediness, of deep and lasting failures. The addicted woman is most often working to do her best, trying to be a good person, a good wife, mother, friend, and worker. Yet she feels bad. She believes herself to be a bad person.

If she thinks she was bad because she was an active addict, then somehow she believes that recovery should make her good. And yet she may continue to feel bad after she becomes abstinent because the shame, guilt, and sense of failure over what she did while actively addicted are so great. She may also feel a deep guilt because she has stopped using and now she is a survivor, one who has started down a new road. She worries about what she has done to others by stopping her addiction: Who has she left behind? Who will be upset by her new knowledge, her new path, and, indeed, her new self? She believes that recovery will make her a good person, but she still doesn't feel like she is a good person. This is what happened to Anne, whom we met in the beginning of this chapter.

When Anne's son, Ken, was twelve years old, he started to get in trouble at school. It was springtime. School was almost out for the year when he was suspended for fighting. Anne knew it had something to do with her. When she drank, her anger bubbled to the surface and found its way out in all sorts of ways. The night before Ken was suspended, Anne had gotten drunk and thrown a plate across the room at her husband, Marty. Ken had walked through the kitchen door at just the wrong moment and the plate almost hit him. Anne suddenly turned on Ken. "Why don't you ever watch where you're going? What are you doing here anyway? You're as bad as your dad. Nobody in this lousy house can pick up a thing. What the hell is wrong with you guys?"

The next morning Anne felt miserable about herself. She could hardly pull her head out from under the covers and face daylight. *What a bad mother I am,* she thought. *What a bad wife. What a bad person.* She vowed she would never lose her temper again. Yet two weeks later she put a dent in the wall by throwing a can of vegetable soup.

Anne quit using and drinking about the time the snow started falling that year. She still felt miserable, but she thought she wasn't going to have to feel miserable about being bad anymore. Imagine her dismay when Ken came home past his curfew on a Saturday evening and she found herself yelling and swearing at him at the top of her lungs. "You stupid, no-good kid!" she yelled before she could stop herself. She stormed out of the house to keep herself from slapping him and walked for a long time in the cool evening air.

What's wrong with me? she despaired. *I still get furious with* my son. *I'm still a bad mother.* She walked until her fingers were like icicles and then headed home, exhausted. Anne had expected that sobriety would mean she would become a good person, but she still felt like a failure.

After Anne had been in recovery for a year, she began therapy to get help with her anger. She began to realize that being sober didn't mean she would never be furious with Ken and Marty. What it did mean was that she could face the fact that she felt furious, and then she could make decisions about how she wanted to act on that feeling.

🌾

Recovery is not a move from bad to good, but from false to real. This is the transformation. The point of surrender and new abstinence represents a letting go of the old self—a false self dominated by a facade of denial, hiding, and desperate attempts to be good and "hold it together." By accepting her loss of control, the woman in recovery opens the door to finding her real, authentic self, the woman she is underneath the layers of defense that have protected her—her false self—perhaps for her entire life. That doesn't mean her real self is "bad" or "good." These categories no longer apply. It is reality, being real, that now guides her rather than her efforts to be good or bad.

🌾

Dependent to Independent or Dependent to Healthy Dependence?
Like the myth that recovery means moving from bad to good, many women think recovery is moving from dependence to self-sufficiency. But there is no such thing as total self-

sufficiency. Self-sufficiency is a partial condition. All human beings are ultimately dependent; all human beings need others on whom they can depend. As the old saying goes, "No man [or woman] is an island." On a physical level, we need others to create new life and to sustain that life. At the most basic level, it takes two to make a baby. It takes even more to form a community that can clothe and feed itself and keep everyone warm and safe. We also need others on an emotional level. We do not outgrow our need for nurture, to be loved and held and understood. Dependence is not a failure, but a normal, healthy part of being human. This is the kind of dependence a woman experiences in recovery.

So let's go back to talking about how the meaning of everything a woman knows changes in recovery and about how she is transformed.

The Truths of Recovery

First, let me expand on the definition of recovery found on page 5: Recovery is a developmental process of finding and building a new self. You will find that the new self is a complex person. You will gain a whole new way of thinking about yourself and about life, a more intricate way of looking at things. It's not black or white, it's not either/or, and it's not good or bad. Instead, this way of thinking recognizes that life is good *and* bad, joyful *and* painful, sweet *and* sour.

Recovery is a more grown-up way of being in the world, and it is filled with complexity. Like all truths, the truths of recovery are mysterious and complex. They are filled with paradoxes—things that seem like they shouldn't both be true at the same time. Things that don't make logical sense. If you look at them logically, they seem absurd. It's what is called "counterintuitive." Everything you thought you were and thought you knew gets reinterpreted and turned around. This makes it hard to hold on to paradoxical truths. Because they seem to contradict logic, they must be experienced to be truly understood. That is one of the reasons it takes a long time to learn these lessons, to learn them in such a way that you know them deep in your bones. You have to take the time to live them in order to truly understand them.

Here are some of the paradoxes of recovery:

1. We are powerless, out of control, and yet, we must take responsibility for being powerless and out of control.
2. All of us need others on whom we can depend; we die without others, and yet we are alone. We can't really connect with others until we've developed a separate self; yet we develop separate selves by connecting with others.

How does it work? How does a woman know that she is powerless and at the same time acknowledge that she had choices in the development of her addiction? How does any woman build a new self on a foundation of powerlessness? How can her strength be anchored in powerlessness? How does a woman come to know that she has a separate self, is independent of others, and, yet, connected to others?

You Are Powerless and You Are Responsible
  for Your Powerlessness
This is one of the most difficult paradoxes to grasp. You come to see yourself straight on, often for the first time, when you acknowledge that you are powerless. As you acknowledge

what really happened, what you did, and how and why you did it, you acknowledge and accept yourself as an agent (someone who can act). You understand that you are a person who made choices that resulted in your utter helplessness. In other words, you have been out of control and you are responsible. With this acceptance of defeat, you come into being.

Many women can accept the first part—being out of control—but not the second part. Many believe that they became out of control because they couldn't help it, because they were the victim of someone else's dominance, aggression, or example. They feel they had no choice because they didn't feel they really existed as a separate person. They only existed through others and to please others. So they feel like addiction happened to them. But as they begin to realize that they do have a separate self, although perhaps muted and stunted, they begin to see that they made choices that led them to become increasingly powerless.

When Anne first went into treatment, she was very clear that she did not have control of either her alcohol and other drug use or of her temper. So all the talk of her being responsible for her addiction was very annoying. After listening to a lecture one evening, she asked the counselor in frustration, "How can you say I'm powerless and that I'm responsible at the same time? It makes no sense."

"Think back, Anne, over the years," her counselor answered. "Think how you came to be in this position. Did someone open your mouth and pour in the gin? When you got mad at Marty, who decided it was easier to pop a pill than to tell him how angry you were? Did Marty make that decision?"

That conversation was repeated in many forms over the next few days, and slowly Anne came to understand how she was responsible for making choices that brought her to this place in her life.

❦

The acceptance of powerlessness and the acceptance of responsibility for being powerless is the great paradox of recovery. As a woman acknowledges herself as an agent, the one responsible for her behavior, she comes into her real self.

❦

You Are Dependent, and You Are Separate and Alone

While all human beings need others, they are also separate and alone. Even while a woman in recovery recognizes that she, like all people everywhere, needs to depend on others, she also recognizes that she needs to develop a self that is separate from others. This is the only way she can know her true self. Recovery is a process of learning who you really are and accepting this person. It's a process of gaining intimate knowledge of your own self. It is the shocking discovery that you are more than your roles and more than your relationships, a discovery that is both liberating and unsettling.

At the same time that you discover you have a separate self, you discover that you are intimately connected to others. In fact, it's only when you have developed a separate self that you can be truly connected with another person. It's a never-ending circle, a mystery. You come to know your real, separate self through connections with other people, and you connect with other people by having a separate self. It's like the proverbial question, "Which came first, the chicken or the egg?"

And ultimately, of course, there is the profound existential reality that we are alone. It is in the quiet, deepest part of ourselves where we think our thoughts and feel our feelings. We can say our thoughts and feelings out loud to others and share them in that way, but others cannot literally think our thoughts and feel our feelings with us.

ᵛᶠ

We are left with the powerful paradox that we need others to survive, and yet we are alone. This is the spirituality of recovery, the knowledge that we have a basic, fundamental need for an "other."

ᵛᶠ

This paradox will become clearer throughout the book as you meet Carole and Blanca, Candace and Sharifa, Mai Lee and Patti, and many other women who struggle to come to terms with their powerlessness and their responsibility, their loneliness, their peaceful aloneness, their strength, and their great capacity to love and be loved.

Recovery as a Developmental Process

Becoming addicted is a developmental process. Many people believe that it happens quickly or that they were always addicted, even born addicted, and were just waiting to live it out. However, no matter how fast or how slowly a woman hooks herself, she still "makes a turn" toward the object of her addiction.

Recovery, too, is a developmental process that takes a long

time. Luckily, you don't undertake this new development alone, and luckily, you can take all the time you need for this radical change. Recovery generally follows certain stages. In part 2 we will look at the developmental stages of addiction and recovery.

PART TWO

A Developmental Process

This book takes a developmental view of addiction. Development usually means forward growth, a process of movement that builds in layers and stages. Here, we'll start by thinking of active addiction as a backward kind of movement, a process of becoming attached to a substance or behavior that interferes with forward, healthy growth and even stops all kinds of normal development.

The person who becomes addicted gets sidetracked and even derailed from a normal developmental path. For example, addiction can slow, distort, or stop all kinds of growth (behavioral, cognitive, emotional, physical, and spiritual) for an adolescent who is just coming into maturity. Addiction can also interfere with a young woman's developing capacity for intimacy and sexuality. It can interrupt an elderly woman's grief or cover up a new mother's anxiety. It can even jump-start a woman's energy, although at great cost to her.

The backward development of addiction involves increasing loss of control. A woman becomes dependent on alcohol, drugs, eating, or spending to take care of her, and eventually the alcohol, drugs, eating, or spending harm her instead. She develops an unhealthy dependence on her "drug of choice," and she then adapts herself to being addicted. She experiences a painful need, or craving, and once she acts on that need, she cannot stop. Being addicted is the repetitive process of acting on impulse to satisfy or quiet internal need, anxiety, or threat.

The process of becoming addicted is one of relinquishment of self. A woman gives up what she knows of her real self and turns instead to constructing a different self. Her "new you" is false, a facade of defenses that rationalize her new "relationship." Being addicted is an ongoing process of backward development, of shutting down and shutting off what is real. Turning this backward slide around is at the heart of the developmental process of recovery. When a woman cannot drink or use or gamble or smoke anymore, when she sees deeply that she has lost control, she may be ready and able to begin a process of recovery.

Recovery, like addiction, is also developmental. The woman must eventually face the loss of herself to her unhealthy dependence. She must face what she has done and what has happened to her as a result of the attachment she made to her addiction. This is a very difficult process. It takes a long time. After having given up her self, she will now begin to reclaim that self and to build a new self.

Recovery development occurs in stages that parallel, metaphorically, human development, from infant to toddler to adolescent to adult. In the next four chapters, we'll follow these stages, looking first at the backward development of addiction, then exploring how the woman makes her separation from her drug of choice and from her active addiction. This separation sets in motion a new development of self. In each stage, the woman in recovery has a primary focus and primary tasks of development, just like the child. As she grows in recovery, she develops a greater complexity of self. Just like a growing child, she can do more, think more, feel more, and integrate it all.

Recovery development is the birth and growth of a healthy self.

Chapter Two

Losing a Self

THE ACTIVE ADDICTION STAGE

M ost of us know that a woman who is an active addict has lost control of her drinking, her use of drugs, or some other compulsive behavior. Most of us also know that she tells herself that she hasn't lost control, that she can control her drinking perfectly well, but she's going to have a drink now because _____.

If you've been an active addict, you know the list of "reasons" to fill in the blank. The kids drove her crazy all day, and she just wants to relax. Her husband was a creep, and she's so angry with him she'll explode if she doesn't have a glass of wine to calm down. If she doesn't drink, she'll never be one of the popular kids, part of the "in crowd" at this school. Scoring drugs on the street keeps her busy, gives her a life. The pills take the edge off the grief she feels since her husband died.

We all know that being an active addict is about loss of control. What everybody doesn't always realize is that there's an even more important loss underneath. This is the loss of self. Slowly but surely, a woman loses track of the person she used to be as she buries her true self in the lies of addiction. She loses what was true about herself. Probably even more important, a woman stops finding out what could be true about herself. She stops developing into a strong, real, grown-up woman. She replaces the course of her natural development with a false self, a grid of lies and defenses that hide or even bury her real self and interrupt her path of normal growth.

Lying to Yourself

You might feel like you were born an addict waiting to happen. And it may be true that you have some genetic vulnerability to addiction that could have sped things up. Sometimes finding yourself in full-blown addiction does feel immediate, particularly if the first drink or hit or pill produced the magic. You found nirvana, and from that point on there was no stopping. Or perhaps becoming addicted may have felt like a slower process. You edged your way down the path, flirting with the beginning cravings you felt, and then you were hooked.

Either way, becoming addicted is a developmental process. You didn't wake up one morning to discover addiction on your skin like a rash you caught unsuspectingly from contact with someone else. No, addiction develops over time, and it involves not only changes in the way you behave but also changes in the way you think: the way you think about drinking, the way you think about yourself, and the way you think about life.

You start to build your sense of self on a false belief, the belief that you can control your drinking or other addictive behavior. This isn't an easy thing to do. Since you really don't have control, you're going to have to lie to yourself in order to believe you're not addicted. You have to tell yourself more and more elaborate lies over time, as evidence to the contrary becomes more compelling and you have to rationalize or explain it away. All your energy goes into pretending.

"Oh what a tangled web we weave, when first we practice to deceive," said the British poet Sir Walter Scott. Scott was talking about the burden that comes to haunt us when we deceive other people—but the burden that comes to haunt us when we deceive ourselves is even worse. Our need to tell ourselves that we can control our addiction becomes the organizing principle for our lives; it dictates everything we say and every move we make. It's a heavy burden, and ultimately it becomes one of the heaviest burdens of all, the burden of emptiness.

Alcohol, other drugs, or whatever substance you are addicted to, becomes the substitute for what is missing in your self. The substance makes you feel like you are powerful. As the initial glow of the bourbon flows into your body, you know that you are cool, happy, interesting, competent, funny, safe. It gives you such a delicious sense of well-being, a sense you can no longer get in any other way. It's false, but it sure feels real. It's quite a bind. You need the substance to feel okay about yourself, but if you admit you need the substance, you can't feel okay about yourself. So you have to pretend, even to yourself.

The result is a smaller, narrower sense of self. You ultimately shut down your deepest experience of self. As a woman who is an active addict organizes her life around her need to drink and her need to pretend that she doesn't need to drink, her life shrinks down. Take Carole, for example.

Carole grew up in upstate New York, the daughter of a lawyer and an engineer. She was very successful in high school. She had a straight 4.0 grade point average, even with advanced physics and calculus. She was extroverted, had a ton of friends, and played basketball. She went to an Ivy League college and was the editor of her school newspaper. Writing, publishing, it was all she ever wanted to do, really. She got a job in New York City when she graduated and in her early thirties became managing editor of a national publication.

Carole came home from work on a hot Tuesday evening. It had been a long day at work, and she was feeling a bit hazy. *That Vicodin might not have been such a good idea this afternoon,* she thought. She was feeling a little uncomfortable with how often she was taking Vicodin these days. Her partner Mary had even been bugging her about it. Still, she knew what she was doing. She used it thoughtfully. On purpose. Only when she knew it would be a good idea.

Carole had a stressful life. Her job was demanding, and some days dealing with all the writers' egos drove her nuts. It was "a challenge," as they say.

She woke up Wednesday morning, got dressed, and started to reach for a Vicodin. *Not today,* she thought. *I'm going to cut back on it.* She struggled out of bed and went to the kitchen. Mary had made coffee before she left for work. As Carole skimmed the newspaper, she began to mentally prepare for the day ahead of her.

She remembered meeting Danielle in the hall the previous day. Danielle had turned her eyes away from Carole, avoiding her. *Jealous,* Carole told herself. *She's not moving up as fast.* Then she thought about Mark and remembered the funny look he gave her after their meeting in the afternoon. *He thinks he's a candidate for my job if I mess up. Hell. No way I'm messin' up.*

She tossed the newspaper aside, went to her bedroom, and put on a midnight blue suit and opal earrings. She poured herself one last cup of coffee for the road but went back into the bathroom before she left to grab the Vicodin. "I've got a hard job," she muttered. "I don't need this stuff, but it can't hurt. I need to stay in charge of those bastards today."

Carole's perceptions are distorted. Danielle had been pre-occupied and hadn't really even noticed Carole as she walked by her in the hall. Mark had given her a funny look at the meeting, but not because he wanted her job. Carole had taken a long time to explain something at the meeting that didn't really matter, and she kept getting distracted. It wasn't really like her. Carole, busy rationalizing her need for Vicodin, couldn't afford to see the self that she had actually presented at the meeting. It was Carole's sharp vision, her ability to understand what was going on around her, that had put her on the fast track in the first place. Now her understanding of who she was and how she fit was getting smaller. Her field of vision was constricting. A woman who is addicted must continually distort her perception of reality in order to keep on believing she has control of her addiction.

Why Women Become Addicted

Asking "why" may not be a useful question for the woman who is still actively addicted. Her answer will likely be one of her rationalizations (the explanations that allow her to keep using, despite all the consequences she now faces). But the woman in recovery can ask why and should ask why. Why did I use? How did I start? What did drinking, or using, or over-eating, or shopping do for me? What did I tell myself? What motivated me to make this turn toward addiction and the loss of my self?

As they reflect back, most women in recovery conclude that drinking was initially positive. Drinking had a purpose. It helped them cope and it helped them adapt. Often, there was a problem to solve or a milestone to celebrate. Drinking or using accomplished the goal. Women drink to get control of themselves, to be better, to feel better, even just to survive. Many women think of their addictive substance or action as an anesthetic that reliably stops what needs stopping: a feeling, a mood, a memory, or an awareness of a painful reality. The addiction works to give women a feeling of control over what is actually uncontrollable within themselves or someone else.

Women may also think of their addictive substance or action as the energizer that gets them going, that fuels a good feeling or mood. Women gamblers and shoppers often report a "high" that comes from the act of betting or spending. This kind of energy also gives them a sense of control. In both cases, to shut down or open up, the woman has a sense that she can be in charge of her internal world. She can be the regulator of her state of mood and mind. "Ah," she says, getting ready to drink. "Soon, all will be well." And it is, for a while.

Drinking gives women the illusion that they can control some problematic aspect of themselves, like being a misfit or not belonging. Some women drink to be able to be mothers. Donella felt that her tranquilizers and sherry gave her the "strength" to be a calm, cool mother to her infant twins and four-year-old. Picturing a little yellow pill or the flow of sherry into her dainty glass gave her stamina through the hard times. She felt the wave of relief with the first sip, and she was able to breathe free. After she'd been sober for several years, Donella could easily say that her supplies of booze and pills helped her control her moods and take the edge off the extremes of emotion she so often felt. Donella had blown up at her kids, so she knew she was capable of hitting them. She lived in terror of herself. That little glass of sherry and that little yellow pill stood between her rages and her kids. Donella could not see the negative consequences of her addiction until she plowed head-on into the garage door with all the kids screaming in the car.

Some women turn to food or spending as a reward for the stress of performing. While they may turn to alcohol or other drugs as well, women often feel more entitled to be out of control with food or spending. A woman can drink, but she will still be faced with scorn and contempt if she is overtly drunk and out of control. Being drunk is an entitlement still reserved for men. Because of this, we often see women's addiction taking different forms.

Sharifa thought she was totally selfless, devoted to everybody else. The only time she could feel okay about taking care of herself, and even really feel that she deserved it, was during her midnight binges. She sat with a carton of ice cream and told herself she deserved this treat. She had given of herself all day and all evening, and now it was her turn. It felt so good eating and eating, but then she felt bad. She eventually came to understand that the treat she really deserved was to stop giving herself away so automatically.

The range of reasons why women become addicted is infinite. Some women become addicted in order to feel and be different; some try to treat anxiety and depression; some want desperately to fit in or to open up; others want to shut down. The woman becomes engaged in a game, and eventually a war, within herself. She is trying to find the perfect amount of scotch, the perfect dose of speed, or the perfect taste of comfort from her chocolate. The "perfect" amount is an elusive goal. She may find it for an instant, and then it's gone. She needs more, but more no longer gives her perfect comfort. It takes her downhill. Becoming addicted almost always starts as positive—it's supposed to solve a conscious or unconscious problem. And then it becomes the problem.

The Process of Becoming Addicted

The process of becoming addicted, and of being addicted, is different from the whys of using. Being addicted is the experience of loss of control, of not being able to stop even when you know you need to stop, when you know you must stop or the world will crash. Addiction starts innocently enough. You drink socially like a lot of other people, and it makes the party go down so much easier. Or you go to the casino on a lark with some friends and hear the ring of bells and clatter of coins as the machine drops twenty quarters into its tin shelf, and for an hour you completely forget that you're supposed to be at work on that night shift you hate. Or you turn to chocolate brownies to stuff your anger when your husband stays late at work for the fourth night in a row and you are stuck alone feeding the kids, cleaning up, and putting them to bed. The thought of the clattering quarters is really appealing the next time you don't feel like working. The next time you're angry at your husband, your mind goes quickly to a soothing ice-cream sundae.

The addiction begins subtly. You don't define the gambling or the alcohol or the excessive food as a need, but as a wish, an interlude. It's occasional. But it moves from subtle to extreme, until you are helpless before the craving. It becomes a painful need for what is now the addictive substance or behavior; you feel like you have to quiet the worry, to soothe the hurt and anger. And you act on it impulsively, over and over again, until it gets in the way of the rest of your life.

Both men and women deny this reality. Like Carole, they

pretend to themselves and everyone else that they are in control, and they end up pretending so frequently that they don't know who they are anymore. They end up losing their sense of self. Here's how it's summed up in *The Handbook of Addiction Treatment for Women*: "Being addicted is the repetitive process of acting on impulse to satisfy or quiet an internal experience that usually includes an emotional threat to the security of self."[1]

Addiction and Trauma

Women sometimes become addicts as they try to soothe the pain of past trauma. When you are traumatized, you feel overwhelmed, both emotionally and physically. Your safety is threatened, and you fear that you will either lose your sense of self and your control over your life or that you may, indeed, lose your life. People who have been traumatized are often haunted by memories of the experience. They may even have flashbacks in which they feel like the experience itself is reoccurring.

Unfortunately, the experience of being utterly overwhelmed, of feeling the safety of the self threatened, is common for women. Many women in recovery, and perhaps even most women in recovery, have been traumatized at the hands of someone who was more powerful than them. They have been physically, sexually, verbally, or emotionally abused. They have felt overpowered or endangered by another. Women who have been traumatized, and especially women who have been

1. S. Brown, "Women and Addiction: Expanding Theoretical Points of View," in *The Handbook of Addiction Treatment for Women: Theory and Practice*, eds. S. L. A. Straussner and S. Brown (San Francisco: Jossey-Bass, 2002), 37.

repeatedly traumatized, seek to quiet the painful memories by drinking or participating in other addictive behaviors. This is not unique to women. Men also seek to tame past traumas by depending on addictive behaviors. They, too, may have been physically, sexually, or emotionally abused. Both men and women have discovered that they can distract and soothe themselves by drinking or by being out of control in many other addictive ways.

Tragically, the behavior they turn to in order to relieve themselves of the pain ends up causing them more pain. The experience of losing control is also traumatic. So the woman who lost control at the hands of another person now loses control at the hands of her addiction. Ironically, the woman becomes the cause of her ongoing trauma. She is her own victim.

Mai Lee was abused as a child. Her uncle lived with her family from the time she was five until she was twelve. At night, when everyone else was sleeping, he would come into her room and fondle her. Her anxiety about this situation caused her to feel sick to her stomach at bedtime. She was relieved when he moved out of the house, and she tried not to think about what had happened. However, as evening approached each day, the anxiety haunted her. She drank a lot during high school, although she managed to keep it from her parents. She succeeded in quelling the anxiety, so much so that she pretty much forgot about it, and her uncle became old news.

After graduating from high school, Mai Lee moved about two hundred miles away from home to attend college. She had a roommate who loved to party, and there were often a lot of people around their apartment late into the evening. Mai Lee found herself feeling increasingly anxious as each evening wore on, but she found that drinking vodka soothed the anxiety. Over time, the vodka made it hard for her to wake up in the morning for classes, and she knew she needed to cut back on her drinking. Each night, however, she found another reason to have just one more drink. Her anxiety began to increase because she knew she needed to cut back on the vodka and she knew, at some level, that she couldn't. She was out of control. The anxiety had reached her stomach, but it hadn't yet reached her consciousness.

Mai Lee experienced childhood trauma, the loss of control she lived with as a victim of another. Her addiction became another traumatic loss of control piled on top of the earlier trauma. Women learn how to live with this addiction, but it's not fun. They bend their lives around like pretzels to avoid knowing how badly they need the alcohol. It is a continual cycle of self-trauma. To interrupt this agonizing cycle, both women and men have to separate from their unhealthy dependence and go back to nurturing and growing the self. In later chapters we will look at how women can practice healthy human dependence, dependence on something that won't hurt them or take control away from them.

What Being an Addict Means to Women

Women were not acknowledged as addicts until the twentieth century, and only in the late twentieth century did a separate field of women and addiction begin to differentiate women's experience of addiction and their needs in treatment from that of men. The research that has emerged has discovered some important things.

Men and women tend to differ in the meanings they attribute to being alcoholic or addicted. For men, being alcoholic or addicted generally means they have failed compared to other men who can drink without losing control. "There are winners and losers; male winners have control. Being a man who can control his drinking is the essence of male power, the essence of competitive edge."[2] Some women attach this same meaning to addiction.

Feeling Like a Loser

As women gained political power in the 1960s, 1970s, and beyond, they fought for equality with men. Many women defined equality as having power in the same way they saw men have power, winning by being in control. This meant not showing vulnerability. Women who were operating out of this framework felt the same need to win, to prove they could control their drinking. For these women, as for so many male addicts, power is control. And if they admit loss of control, they are no longer powerful. They lose. Of course, it is an illusion for women just as it is for men. While women may feel they are "at war" with men for a claim to equal power over their ability to drink, they are actually "at war" with themselves. These women experience addiction as a power struggle against loss of control within the self—drinking, using other drugs, overeating, overspending, gambling. They are losers in a battle for power.

Power is also related to competition. Men tend to see their need to control their drinking as a masculine contest—man to man, who can outdrink the other? This is evidence of male power, male virility. Sometimes women have the same competitive drive—the need to win over someone else. Many

2. S. Brown, "Women and Addiction: Expanding Theoretical Points of View," in *The Handbook of Addiction Treatment for Women: Theory and Practice,* eds. S. L. A. Straussner and S. Brown (San Francisco: Jossey-Bass, 2002), 46.

women feel compelled to join the men in drinking and drug-ging as a way to break through the glass ceiling, or simply to be and feel equal in the workplace. Or women can feel more aggressive, more powerful, more able to speak, if they've got an excuse. The old phrase "it was the alcohol talking" gives women permission.

Feeling Inadequate

More often women see their addiction as meaning they are a failure in their relationships. The failure is not in a battle for power this time, but a failure to perform up to standards. They have not performed well in their roles as wives, girlfriends, mothers, or partners.

So many women define themselves by their role. Their value arises from what they do for others. They often measure themselves against the way other women are carrying out these roles and believe they don't "measure up," they are not as successful in the role of wife, girlfriend, mother, or partner. Or they may feel they have failed because they are not as sat-isfied and accepting in these traditional roles as other women seem to be. And if they are not doing what they think they should be doing for others, they are failures. They are not measuring up to the ideal they hold of the role they are sup-posed to play. When they acknowledge that they are addicted, there is often a great deal of shame attached to what they see as their failure as women who have not behaved as women should behave.

Getting Ready for Recovery

Although women become addicted for many reasons and may attach different meanings to the fact that they are addicted, the experience of loss of control is the same as it is for men. So, too, is the process of recovery. The woman sacrifices her self and her relationship with herself in the service of maintaining an active addiction. The key to recovery is to reclaim her self, minus the active addiction, or to find and develop a healthy self for the first time.

*

The path to the end of active addiction is rugged. It is so difficult, so frightening, and so unpredictable that many women don't make it. Frequently the problem is that they don't really want re-covery; they still want to get control.

*

The end of active addiction is indeed the end of the fight to get control. Women in AA and other Twelve Step programs call this end of the road "hitting bottom" or "surrender." The woman says, "I am an alcoholic/I am an addict. I have lost control." This is often a momentous occasion, a time of great desperation and resistance, sometimes a time of flashing in-sight or spiritual awakening. It is what many women believe will be their death. They will come face to face not only with the reality that they have lost control, but with the equally harsh truth that they cannot regain control. Getting control is not to be.

For many women this is death. But for the woman who ac-cepts her loss of control and her inability to regain it, this death becomes something quite different than she feared. It will be the death of her false self, the collapse of her denial, rationalizations, delusions, and illusions, all the defenses that provided the false scaffolding that became her self. The end of the road of active addiction is the death of the false self that covered a real person with real needs, longings, vulnerabilities, strengths, and talents.

Along with this experience of defeat, the woman also comes to see that she does not know how to stay abstinent, and she asks for help. Asking for help frees her from the prison of her self-sufficiency and isolation and opens the way for the birth of her new self. She now has the opportunity to find and grow the woman she was underneath it all, and the woman she can be. Welcome to recovery.

Chapter Three

Recovery Shock

THE TRANSITION STAGE

Imagine the trauma of transition that a newborn baby experiences as she enters the world. Imagine the change in her environment from shadows to bright light, from muted sounds to sharply delineated noises. Imagine the intensity of her feelings and her frantic need for soothing, holding, and a parent to care for her. The overwhelming sense of chaos. This is what the beginning of recovery is like. Shock. Moving from active addiction to abstinence is like being born all over again.

In this chapter we will look first at the chaos of feeling and thought that greets a woman when she awakens from addiction, and next at how she can cope with this. Let's begin with Geri.

Geri had been sober for a full week, since the day she could not wake up to take care of her kids, two-year-old Willy and three-year-old Molly. John, her husband, had been out of town, and she had gone to bed in a blackout. The next morning she found Molly standing on a chair by the kitchen counter with grape jelly smeared everywhere. Willy was balancing on the same chair dipping his fingers in and out of the jelly jar and licking them. There was a butcher knife nearby and a glass broken on the floor. That was the moment Geri decided she would not drink again.

She had gone to a meeting each of the last five days. She hung on each day until John got home from work, and then she quickly left for her meeting. But John traveled for his work a couple days every week, and now he was gone and she hadn't been able to find a babysitter for tonight's meeting. *I can manage this one night*, she thought. *I have to manage.*

The kids were finally in bed. *I can handle this*, she repeated to herself. *I can handle this.* Geri snuck a look at the children, then headed for the bathtub, looking for soothing and comfort. She lay back in the warm water and closed her eyes. The first image that rose in front of her was of herself, grabbing her son and sitting him roughly in his chair at dinner. *What a miserable excuse for a mother I am*, she thought. Her next thought was of a glass of gin. She swore aloud and then burst into tears. She held her face in her hands, thoughts crashing against each other. *Idiot. You're supposed to be happy now. What's wrong with you? You want a damn gin. Why isn't John home like a husband's supposed to be? What a jerk he is. He's the one who's been after me to stop.* Then she stopped herself. *No, no, no, no. Not John's fault. I'm the jerk. I'm the jerk who wants the gin.*

The warm water gave her no comfort. She stood up abruptly, wrapped herself in a towel, and headed to the kitchen for a bowl of ice cream. She added chocolate chips. Then butterscotch. Then pecans. She finished the bowl in five minutes. *Fat cow*, she said to herself.

Geri headed back upstairs, turned on the television in her bedroom, and slipped into a nightgown. She tuned into a detective show, but it was hard to pay attention. Her body and mind were both restless. She turned off the show and grabbed her novel. She would read herself to sleep. As she read, her eyelids grew heavy and she became semi-aware of entering that blessed twilight zone. She let the book slip from her hand.

"Mommy!" Geri's eyes popped open to find her daughter standing by her bed, tugging at her arm. Startled out of her half-sleep, Geri felt the cry like an assault. Lights, little prickling flashes of lights, fired in front of her, and she wanted to reach out and slap her daughter. "Leave me alone!" she shouted. One more time she buried her face in her hands and cried. She was shocked by the misery, terrified that she couldn't do this.

Some women are lucky. They experience new abstinence as a wonderful thing, a huge relief. But they are the exception. Most newly abstinent women are like Geri: They feel like they're getting worse instead of getting better. And for many women, it's not just a feeling; it's the truth.

Feeling Again

After they stop drinking, most women feel terrified of what will happen, full of guilt and shame, and so alone. It's like losing a husband or partner, or a best friend. Someone on whom they depend. They've experienced a death of sorts. Like the woman whose husband of many years dies. A week later she reads a book and looks up to tell him about the passage she's read. She says his name before she remembers. She wakes in the night and reaches out to feel for him. And then she remembers. Over and over she feels the impact of the loss, the disorientation, the panic. The shock of recovery is the shock of profound loss and the experience of many new and painful feelings.

With or without addiction, women often feel painful contradictions in their lives. They grow up learning that they are defined by their relationships and what they do for others. They are mothers first, wives first, friends first. And only second are they themselves. Women often feel guilty when they have desires for themselves, when they want time for themselves, and when they have personal aspirations. They're caught in a bind. They feel like failures as mothers if they put their careers or themselves first, and they feel like failures in the world if they sacrifice themselves for their families. They don't have a whole self. Some women escape the horrible conflict of these contradictions by putting everything out of mind—out of awareness—by softening the sharp pain of failures and needs and wants by being addicted.

And then, they are newly abstinent. And oh, do they start to feel. When women in recovery take away their anesthetic, or their energizer—the alcohol, the other drugs, the robotic eating and spending, or the obsessive, all-consuming passion for controlling another—what do they have left?

When Carole flushed away her Vicodin, she cried. She cried every day for three weeks. Getting up each morning was the most painful thing she ever did. Even the sun coming through her window accused her of idiocy.

Mai Lee's grades dropped to Cs and worse in all her classes the semester she got sober. She couldn't listen in class. Half the time she couldn't even go to class. Depression hit her so hard she gave up getting out of bed for a week. Fortunately, her sponsor steered her to a therapist.

By the time Donella got sober her kids were almost grown, and the grief she felt about the time she had lost with them stayed with her every minute of every hour of every day, day after day. It was months before she was able to forgive herself and even longer before the grief lessened.

Sharifa felt another kind of recovery shock. Some women don't feel shame about their out-of-control behaviors because they think they're doing good things. They don't understand that they have a problem. Sharifa was a very kind woman and always available to her friends. She was such a good listener that people were always calling when they were upset about something and needed a friend. Sharifa liked this about herself; she liked being a compassionate person, and when the phone rang, she went on duty. In fact, she didn't think she really had a choice. It was her primary job to be a good listener. At the same time, she found she couldn't get her own projects done. So when she hung up the phone, before she let herself feel annoyed, she'd open up the refrigerator door and reward herself with a snack. She found herself putting on a lot of weight, but she felt good about the kind of person she was.

Since women like Sharifa are only trying to please, they can't grasp that things they are doing are "wrong," things like eating constantly, driving up their blood pressure, and causing themselves other physical problems. The very fact that these women are addicted comes as its own shock. Yet these women, too, feel the shock and pain of denied feelings as their addictive coping mechanism is removed. Sharifa moved from binging to bulimia before she was able to quit using food as a drug. Every time she looked in the mirror she cringed at what a hideous person she was.

Women in the shock of new recovery are left with themselves, the woman underneath the false self of the addiction and her identity as a role-bound female. As they awaken, they find that the feelings they used to have—feelings they wanted to escape in the first place—are there waiting for them.

Sharp Feelings

New recovery is painful on several levels. First, newly recovering women must deal with the normal feelings that most women have but which they have buried under addiction. Second, they have to face the ambivalence they feel as they bring their own recovery needs into balance with meeting the needs of others. Third, they experience shame and guilt, loss, sadness, and other difficult feelings as they face the sometimes outrageous, irresponsible, and even dangerous things they did during their addiction. Fourth, they may find themselves threatened by new, or more intense, memories of trauma during their childhood and adult life.

Unfortunately, many women don't know that it's normal to feel a full range of emotions in sobriety, from anxiety to sadness to pleasure. What's more, they don't want this kind of "normal." They want to feel better. They don't want to hear that this is what you get when you stop using.

*

It's very hard to hear that recovery is about learning to accept problems, conflicts, and emotional pain as normal and then learning different ways to cope. Women may conclude that they are doing something wrong if they are having problems in recovery. Quite the contrary. The fact that they are having problems and emotional pain is a sign that they are in recovery.

*

Added to the normal pain and confusion of their everyday lives is the shame of things they did when they were addicted. Shame is what Geri felt when she thought about her young children alone in the kitchen with sharp knives and broken glass. It's deeply painful for newly abstinent women to acknowledge what they did or didn't do while addicted.

They also feel guilty and selfish about taking time away from their friends and family for recovery. How does a woman manage the opposing poles of guilt now that she is sober? Maybe she didn't take care of her kids when she was using, and doesn't it just make it even worse that she's focusing on her recovery instead of taking care of them now? Maybe she did take care of them and can't bear to turn her attention away. A woman in new recovery often feels guilt for what she did while drinking and guilt for what she's doing now by being sober: guilt for failing and guilt for succeeding, guilt for existing. Isn't she the cause of everything that has ever gone wrong anywhere?

When you take away your anesthetic, or your energizer, you will begin to feel and to see what life is really like, including the bad and the good. When the artificial feelings produced by alcohol or other drugs are gone, you will experience many frightening feelings. You may feel anxious and depressed. You may feel sad or ashamed. Guilty. Unworthy. Angry. Even feeling good can cause anxiety. Feeling good can seem out of control, or it can be the signal of a binge about to start. Good or bad, you will probably feel confused. Most of all, you may feel terrified.

Finally, women who have been traumatized often feel deeply troubled in the beginning of recovery and, indeed, well into recovery. Newly abstinent women may find these feelings suddenly are not buried or disguised. We'll look at this again later in the chapter.

No Feelings

In addition to having many feelings, it is also normal not to feel anything in early recovery. You may stay numb for a while. You focus on the new behaviors of recovery and you listen. You think a lot and you make connections. Things start to make sense. You know you're an addict. But you don't feel. Not for a long time. Whether you feel a lot, feel a little, or feel nothing at all, it is normal. You just don't want to start using in order to stop the feelings or in order to start them.

How Do I Cope?

If you are like many other women in early abstinence, you feel inadequate, maybe even dumb. How did you get yourself into this predicament? And what do you do now? How do you stay away from your drug of choice and every other drug too? How do you focus on yourself one day at a time? What self? How do you feel deserving of sobriety, of what you now hear are the "promises," when you feel like you're abandoning your family by going out to meetings and putting this focus on yourself? How do you tell your family that you need to stop drinking and that you need meetings when they don't think anything is wrong? Or when they're so angry they don't want to stick around while you get well? Most of all, how do you survive each moment and each day when the pain is so great and you are so scared?

The Baby Stage

The newly abstinent woman is very much like a baby in the sense that she doesn't know how to stop her addictive impulses and behaviors, she doesn't know what to do with her intense feelings, and she doesn't know the words to express any of this. She often feels like a bundle of raw nerve endings, agitated and full of panic. Like an infant, full of sensation, instinct, and impulse, she needs help. She needs instruction in simple, concrete terms about what to do next and time to learn how to take one baby step at a time.

Form a Healthy Attachment

The transition from active addiction to recovery begins with a new attachment, the cornerstone foundation of new development. A baby has to be attached to a primary caretaker in order to grow, and this is typically the mother, is somewhat less often the father, but can also be a grandparent, aunt, or other adult. Attachment is food for the baby's soul. The baby can't develop without it. The trust and connection are what allow the baby to learn that soothing is possible, that there is safety in the world, and that she can cry for help and help will come. Attachment nurtures and grows the neural connections that create a fully functioning brain. A baby can get all the food she needs, but if the baby is offered no one to attach to, she will wither. The attachment to the mother builds, and in turn, the capacity for the baby, and then the child, and then the teenager, and then the adult, to have healthy relationships with other people. Human beings are fundamentally dependent on others to develop, not only physically, but emotionally as well.

Similarly, recovery is built on attachment to a nurturing "parent." Initially, the attachment may be to a treatment program, Twelve Step meetings, or a woman's own concept of a higher power. This attachment is the foundation of healthy dependence and a healthy separate self. It is also the foundation of what will become a healthy spirituality. A woman lets go of her deep attachment to alcohol, of her relationship to her substance, and she shifts that attachment to abstinence and the resources that support it. In the beginning she will rely in a simple, concrete way on others for support. Over time, a more complex and deeply trusting relationship with a higher power grows within her as she matures. The woman's new attachment to recovery resources is *not* to her partner, nor to anyone with whom she already has a close, personal relationship (such as a family member or friend). She has to have a new primary dependency relationship outside of her family. And it is this new relationship to AA or other recovery resources that will offer her the "other" that will be her guide to new self-development.

The Eighteen-Second Rule, or Body Learning

Let's carry the baby analogy a bit further. In early abstinence a woman, like a baby, will have strong impulses and anxieties, and also like a baby she will need instant attention given to these feelings. A woman in recovery needs to focus on quieting her impulses and anxieties with new behaviors. And she must respond instantly. She must substitute a new abstinent behavior (make a call, run to a meeting, drink a Coke, take a walk) for the old addicted behavior. These substitutes will redirect her intense craving to drink or act out another addiction. By quickly changing her behavior, she can gain a sense of quiet. This is also referred to as "behavioral abstinence." Let's look at Patti for an example of how this works.

Patti, who had been abstinent for four weeks, dropped off her five-year-old daughter at afternoon kindergarten. She was on her way home to start the laundry before she went to her meeting when she noticed she was driving by an Italian café, a little place where she often went with some of the other women in the neighborhood who had little kids. She loved the Chianti at Mario's, and suddenly she wanted a drink. She wanted a drink so badly she could literally taste it on her tongue. The smooth, dry taste of it swirling in her mouth. *Glass of wine. Glass of wine.* The sweet sense of relaxation spreading through her body. *Glass of wine. Deep red wine.*

She was terrified. *I want this to last,* she thought. *I've made it through a whole month.* Then she remembered something she heard from Loretta the second night she went to a meeting. "An impulse to drink only lasts for eighteen seconds. If you can hang on for eighteen seconds, you'll make it through the craving." Patti pulled over to the side of the road and fished frantically through her purse for her cell phone, counting as she did. "One . . . two . . . three . . . four . . . five . . ." Loretta's number was programmed into her cell phone. Which number did she have to push now? Oh yeah, 12. She listened to the ring of the phone, counting again. "Nine . . . ten . . . eleven . . ."

"Loretta. Thank God you're there. I'm in front of Mario's and I want to go in for wine."

Patti made it through the impulse. Eighteen seconds felt like an eternity to her as she waited out the intense craving. But it passed. An impulse may last a lot longer than eighteen seconds, or it may feel like a lot longer. The key here is that Patti put into immediate action the behavioral substitutes she needed. It is the redirection of the impulse—taking action in a new way—that helps end the craving.

The Toddler Stage

Head Learning

As a baby moves into the toddler stage, she begins to acquire a new kind of learning. She begins to pick up language, which builds the foundation for understanding and forming ideas. Similarly, the woman born newly into abstinence begins what is called cognitive learning. She listens to others tell the stories of what they did in the past and what they do now. She begins to hear a new language, the language of recovery, and thus, like a toddler, begins to form her new self and her new identity around the acceptance of her addiction. She comes to know the words "I am an alcoholic" or "I am an addict" and builds her new, strong sense of self on this foundation.

When Patti got to her meeting, she began to feel calmer as she listened. She remembered when she first started coming to this meeting, the words sounded like gibberish. But today they made sense to her. When Joan spoke of her intense, blinding need to use again, it made sense to Patti. And when Joan talked about calling her sponsor, taking a walk, doing something to substitute for the compulsion to drink, Patti connected. The words almost felt like music. She felt held, and even rocked, by the growing familiar sounds of people talking in the AA meeting and the relief of understanding what they meant.

Heart Learning

As a woman feels the attachment to sober people, imitates their behavior, identifies through their modeling, and understands through their stories, she begins to grow up again, this time for real. Here begins the paradox of how she finds her self through others. And here begins the learning about the self, the reclaiming and development of the person she is. As her addiction no longer smothers her real feelings, she can begin to recognize the emotions of her real self. It is only through allowing yourself to feel your authentic feelings that you will begin to know who you really are.

A Focus on Self

Your main job at this point is to tolerate the shock of recovery and to hold your focus on yourself. The task of focusing on yourself may sound simple, but it is incredibly complex. How do you focus on yourself and your recovery when you don't have a self yet?

First, and this bears repeating, you need to practice substituting abstinent behaviors, such as phoning new friends, going to meetings, and taking a walk if you feel a craving to return to addictive behavior. You also need to listen to the stories of other women who identify as addicts who have lost control. As you listen, you come to recognize, "that is me," "I did that," "I thought like that." The more you listen, the more your new sense of self begins to take shape. It's based on reality—the reality of what you did, what you thought, and what you felt.

In the meantime, you need to tolerate the anxiety of not knowing—not knowing what you feel about people and things, not knowing yourself well enough to trust that what you think and feel is really what you think and feel. It's normal to develop a self based on what you learn from those around you and what you discover on your own. But women who are addicted lose the ability to tell the difference between what others feel and want from their own feelings and desires. They discount their own feelings. In recovery, you will still learn by listening to others, but you will also work on noticing what you feel and think. This is called finding the boundary of your self. You focus on finding the self that is separate from others. Even though you are identifying with others, you are concentrating on learning what is true for you.

Fitting in Family and Friends

The task of focusing on yourself is difficult when you have so many other people who need and may demand your attention. You have to deal with the reality of your life with others, and you will likely feel confused and conflicted about just what is most important.

You will have a new primary dependency relationship outside of your family: your attachment to AA and other recovery resources. So is it any wonder that spouses often feel their newly recovering wives are in the throes of an affair? You have to separate to some degree from your family in order to pursue healthy self-development. When women begin to put this focus on themselves, it frequently becomes a source of tremendous difficulty with others early on in the recovery process. It brings on new tension at home about what is to be the primary focus: Are you to put your recovery first, or does it come after your family's needs?

⁂

Often in early abstinence, those close to you hope that you will get things under control and return to being the woman you used to be. You may have seen your behavior as self-sacrificing, but that doesn't mean they did. They may wish that you would just "get it together." As you feel this pressure, it is altogether too easy to feel drawn back into putting others first.

⁂

Sometimes the shift to a helpful outside relationship is a welcome relief for family. They are supportive, happy, and proud. But sometimes this shift outside of family brings anxiety, fear, and tension. As much as partners and friends may have longed for recovery, the reality of the woman's new attention to her self and to her new supports can bring feelings of loss, abandonment, betrayal, and jealousy to those close to her.

After Geri's first week of sobriety, she got herself into treatment. She went during the day for four weeks. The children had been in part-time day care, and she was able to extend it to full days for the four weeks of treatment. After treatment, Geri found a continuing care group that met at 6:00 P.M. on Thursday evenings. Thursday night was also John's poker night. When Geri told him he had to cancel his poker night, he was really upset.

"You know I want to support you, Geri," he said. "But how can you ask me to give up my poker night? I've been doing this for two years. I work hard all week. I need this time."

All along John had been telling Geri to do what she needed to do. But she had a hunch that he meant she should do what she needed to do as long as it didn't inconvenience him. This turned out to be true. She didn't know whether to feel angry or guilty. She didn't argue. Instead she spent half an hour calling around until she found a babysitter, and she went late to her meeting. But she couldn't keep spending that kind of money every Thursday.

By the time she got to the meeting she was seething. Then humiliated. Then seething. *I'm supposed to talk about stuff when it's hard,* she reminded herself. The others in the group were very supportive. They talked about the kinds of adjustments they had gone through, and they suggested she sit down with John and together come up with a schedule that would work for both of them.

Geri was faced with a need for a serious compromise right away. She gathered up her courage when they got home from their respective activities. Talking with John turned out to be easier than she thought. John understood her frustration. They talked it over, and John suggested he ask his folks if they'd come over on Thursday evenings and take care of the children.

It was important that Geri did not sacrifice her recovery to make John feel okay. At the same time, she couldn't automatically expect that he would sacrifice his life either. She could not suddenly expect everyone to do things her way or to put her recovery ahead of their own needs. Yet this is exactly what she wanted. At this point she didn't understand compromise at all. She still thought that somebody wins and somebody loses. Now it was her turn to win because she was supposed to be first. Geri learned about compromise early on. She also learned that family and relationship issues from the past and present would be right there to hit her in the face. You can drive yourself crazy trying to sort it all out, especially if you want everyone to be happy. As you struggle with all of these difficult relationship issues early on, remember *you must put your recovery first.*

Once again, it's not all or nothing. If you have young children, you must think of them, of course. You must be sure they are safe and protected as you turn to your own new growth. And you need to develop a balance between meeting the needs of others, both family and friends, and meeting your own needs. Resolving this tension will be an ongoing issue in the present, and it will be complicated by your experiences from the past.

How do you do this? You keep your recovery focused by getting help. This attention to self is easiest if your family and friends are understanding and supportive. And, in fact, your self-development works best if the other important people in your life are engaged in the same process. You need support and so do your children. So does your husband or partner. Everybody needs support to sustain this kind of monumental change. Everybody is going to grow; everybody is going to change. It's scary, but a focus on self for each person offers the best possibility for healthy couples growth and healthy family growth down the road.

Recovery and Trauma

Many women who are addicted have suffered severe childhood traumas or have lived with severe trauma as adults. Many identify as adult children of alcoholics or as codependents (women who learned in their childhood families to sacrifice themselves to meet the unhealthy needs of their families). While virtually all women who have learned the social and cultural roles of self-sacrifice find it tough to know their separate "selves," it is particularly hard for women who have suffered trauma at the hands of another to separate their real selves from the false selves they developed in their childhood families.

These women grew up with alcoholic parents or with other disturbances and difficulties—verbal and physical abuse, sexual abuse—that could not be acknowledged or dealt with directly. They grew up with secrets, the binding glue of traumatic families. Denying these awful traumas, while having to endure them, leads directly to a loss of self and to the creation of a false self. The child goes into emotional hiding. She buries her real self as she adapts herself to the needs and realities of her traumatic world. She gives up her own individual, autonomous development in the service of belonging to, and defending, her addicted, disturbed, and traumatic childhood family. This kind of early family system reinforces the importance of her selflessness.

When this woman enters recovery, she is often shocked by the reality of her own loss of control and by the sudden return of memory, memory of the realities and traumas of her childhood that she isn't supposed to have. She may have a very hard time staying sober if the past intrudes too quickly. Ironically, recovery itself becomes a trauma for these women. If you find yourself shocked by the return of traumatic memories, it is important to get extra help. Find a psychotherapist who can help you cope with your responses to these memories.

Some women feel and remember slowly, protected from overwhelming pain by a hazy awareness and an intense focus on new behavior and the nuts and bolts of staying sober. These women are protected until they have enough sobriety to tolerate the pain.

If you have lived a life in which trauma eroded your sense of self, you will begin to find your real self in recovery. You will find your real self as you remember and unwind the knotted umbilical cords of painful relationships. You will recognize how you adapted yourself by default to an unhealthy family system or relationship, how loss of self has been your definition. Until now. Now, as you begin to feel comfortable with your new behaviors and stronger identity as an addict, you will take your next developmental step into early recovery.

Relapse

Before we move on to talk about the next stage of development, I want to spend a little time on relapse. Returning to active addiction after a period of abstinence is not unusual, nor even abnormal. This happens sometimes because women haven't really "hit bottom" yet, and sometimes because the pull of the addiction overcomes them.

Many women move back and forth from active addiction into abstinence until they stabilize in solid abstinence. This fluctuation is called "fits and starts." Some women try out abstinence before they hit bottom. They make a test run to see if they can stand it. But they haven't really made it to recovery yet. They don't really understand or accept that they have lost control. It's more like taking a break from active addiction. This was the case for Donella. As she told her story at a meeting, she said:

> I used to say I was relapsing. Not so. I never hit bottom, I never really accepted that I had lost control, and I never wanted to stay stopped. Being dry was my time out, my temporary effort at control.

Others hit bottom, move into recovery, and then teeter like baby fawns on wobbly legs, finally stumbling back to using. These are women who relapse. They had experienced surrender, shifting from a belief in control to an acceptance of loss of control, and they had started to alter their behavior. Next they wobble and their legs collapse. Hopefully this is a temporary reversal, and they pull themselves back up again, back into abstinence and another try at accepting and living with the reality of their loss of control.

Warning of Relapse or Pain of Recovery?

How will you know if you're about to relapse? You might not. If you fear you're about to relapse, what matters is that you intensify your focus on yourself. You intensify your attachment to your recovery and your recovery resources.

Many women fear that their new behaviors won't hold them. The new thinking and language of recovery makes no sense, and they're scared they will be overwhelmed with feelings or that memory will be unbearable. And so they don't make a deep attachment to recovery to begin with, or they let their strong attachment loosen. They decrease attendance at meetings, stop calling a sponsor, and begin to think that they're different, that they aren't as bad as some of these women they now know. Donella's story continued:

> I bounced back and forth, in recovery, out of recovery. I felt like such a failure. I made a mess of drinking and now I couldn't get recovery. I relapsed every time I got sixty days. It was like Pavlov's bell. At day fifty-nine I could taste it. Finally I dreamed that I miscounted and it was day sixty-one. I was full of guilt. How had I failed to drink? I woke up and felt depressed. I knew I had broken a rule: I wasn't supposed to be successful. I wasn't supposed to be sober. But here I was. This time I made it to day sixty-one and have been sober ever since.

If you relapse, then get back on the horse and ride again. Whether this is your first attempt at recovery, or second, or fifth, the beginning of recovery is almost always a rough ride. It can't be otherwise. If you have a strong attachment to recovery, to AA, to your new identity as an alcoholic, you will use this foundation as the ground on which you do the hard developmental work. You will struggle, like an infant and toddler, to negotiate the early developmental tasks and to build, layer upon layer, a new, healthy self. Your job is to stay attached, to question any loosening of your program of recovery. When you can't tell what is what, when you are confused about whether you are struggling with the normal conflicts and tensions of healthy growth or whether you are bound for a relapse, you strengthen your basic recovery actions and hold on. Then, as you get stronger again, you will move from wobbling to standing, from crawling to baby steps, and on to walking.

In summary, when you stop your drinking or other addiction, you arrive metaphorically as a naked infant in the new world of recovery, you find yourself overwhelmed with an array of intense and confusing feelings. You feel anxious and uncertain about what has happened to you and what you are supposed to do now. Like all babies, you need to form a strong bond with a nurturing "other" such as AA meetings and other recovery resources. You also discover that you must immediately substitute new behaviors for old cravings and listen carefully to others who have made it through this difficult time. You feel like an infant in a grown-up body. You know you need help, but you're afraid of help at the same time.

Nevertheless, you continue to attend meetings, and you learn the language of recovery. You keep your focus on yourself. You make sure your children are safe, and you encourage your family to get the help they, too, need in the recovery process. But you keep your focus on yourself. And one day you will wake up and realize that you are no longer in a constant, low-grade panic.

Chapter Four

The Growth of a New Self

The Early Recovery Stage

A bell doesn't ring to signal this next stage of growth, but you know you're there when you have an impulse to drink and you can think about it, watch it, turn it around in your mind, and then take a recovery action. You've reached early recovery when you can trust that eighteen seconds will pass.

Early recovery brings a lessening of intense impulse, a lessening of that strong physical need to do something instantly or you'll go crazy. It doesn't mean you won't ever feel this kind of need again or that you stop paying attention to recovery behaviors. It is still a time of action. But painful craving is no longer the focal experience of your inner self. Now you can turn your attention to active learning rather than to an instant coping action to quiet an impulse.

Growing a Self

The key work of early recovery is developing a strong sense of your inner self. Reclaiming and developing a self is a process that takes time. Early recovery is the chance to grow up all over again, so time is your great friend. If you try to go too fast, you can miss important developmental building blocks, leaving you with holes in your new self. In a certain sense, the woman who skips developmental work in recovery can end up with a learning disability. You'll have a handicap if you rush too fast. Yet it may be hard to slow down. You're excited about learning as much as you can, as fast as you can, and you want to "get there," to be grown-up.

Early recovery is also a period of intense change. You will continue to focus on your abstinent behaviors, of course, strengthening your instant responses to impulse or to anxiety. But by this time you know how to move quickly to get out of danger and to get support. This security allows you to do the work of finding out who you are, to think about your self. Along with this new ability to think comes ever more feelings, another reason you may want to hurry up and get there. You want to quiet the inner turmoil. You've got a full plate.

Early recovery is all about reality, finding and developing a self that is real. You'd think that would be simple, that it's easy to know what is real. But that's not the case. Knowing what is real is about as hard as anything in recovery because before you became sober, you couldn't know what was real. Reality could not be seen or felt. Reality was taboo. That's why you needed a false self. The woman in early recovery is faced with the daunting and confusing task of reclaiming a self she can barely remember and maybe never knew.

How Do I Find a Self?

How do you find a self that's been put away in the closet for years? How do you grow a self that stopped developing when you were a child? You may feel utterly confused about how to begin this search. Fortunately, the answer is within you. You find your self again, and nurture the growth of that self, by paying attention. It will be a new sensation, paying attention to what you're feeling and wanting. And you won't always know in the beginning. You may be so used to not paying attention to what you feel and want that you don't even recognize it. But you will learn by doing it. You will learn by learning the language of recovery, by listening and speaking the language of the self, by being in relationships with other people, and by continuing to notice and assert yourself.

The Maturing Child

Language Development

In developmental terms, an infant can only communicate her needs by inarticulate cries. To indicate hunger, an infant roots her head against a mattress or a bottle or a breast and makes sucking sounds and motions with her lips. As she becomes a toddler, her instinct for language develops and she begins to learn words. In the more mature stages of childhood, she increases her ability to use language, both to understand her world and to meet her needs. Language acquisition is a milestone for children, just as standing and learning to walk are milestones. Language is the great mediator, the bridge of delay, between impulse and action. Language gives the young child a vocabulary to express her inner self in a new way.

In the early days of recovery, a woman is like the young but maturing child in her increasing ability to use language for learning. Most children love the sound of a new word, and they love to repeat words and chants (a ritual that is also fundamental to the Twelve Step process and experience). Words can take children out of fear. They allow kids to tame invisible, frightening monsters and thus to transform what had been terrifying. Words also give kids a sense of security and competence in acknowledging, naming, and mastering what had been unknown or hidden. So before a child has language, when she is frightened by the night, she cries and needs her parent to reassure her. At the next stage of development, she can use language to think, *I'm scared of monsters.* She can use words she has learned with her parent to calm herself. *There are no monsters under the bed* or *The night doesn't hurt me.*

※

In recovery, the word mastery *does not mean a return to "control." Instead, it means an ability to cope with life's challenges; it means acceptance, tolerance, and integration. It doesn't mean a woman controls her fear so that she never feels like there are monsters under her bed. It means that she recognizes and accepts that the fear of monsters is part of life and she can cope with it.*

※

In other words, the woman learns that naming takes away the power of an impulse, that talking about how and what she feels reduces her tension.

She also learns that naming adds new feelings, the emotions that belong to all the realities she so carefully denied. She uses language to reflect on herself, her past, and her present. As she gives names to her feelings, they become more real.

The language of recovery makes this possible. The power of language provides a sense of distance and safety that allow her to feel more, not less, of the past and more of the present.

This distance in turn gives her the internal space to pause and reflect, something she could never allow before. The use of language teaches her about her new identity and developmental needs. The ritual use of this language reinforces her identity and growth, helping the woman to integrate her new learning into her self. She says, "Hi, my name is Tess. I'm an alcoholic." She hears the realities and the values of recovery like a mantra that wraps and holds her steady while they become part of her very being. Let's look at an example of how this new language promotes mastery in early recovery.

Anne got a call from school saying her son, Ken, had skipped second hour. "Do you know where he is?" they asked. She wondered how they expected her to know. What did they think she was, psychic or something? She thought he was done with this crap, and now she was going to have to face it all over again. She walked into the bathroom to grab some hand lotion and noticed that her hand of its own volition had gone to the back of her cosmetics drawer. It's where she used to keep her Xanax, but it was not there anymore. So she wheeled around and opened the medicine cabinet. Somewhere she had some leftovers from a prescription for codeine.

Then the words from last night's meeting appeared as a gift. *Easy does it.* She took a deep breath and rehearsed to herself: *One step at a time.* She told herself, *Make a call. Slow down.* She turned and walked out of the bathroom, repeating over and over, *Easy does it . . . Easy does it . . . Easy does it . . . Easy does it.* She went to the kitchen and decided she would make herself a cup of tea. Even as she did so, the intensity of the drive toward oblivion lessened. She found herself smiling. *Huh. This slogan stuff actually works,* she thought. Not that she didn't still want the Xanax. But her hand wasn't darting toward the bottle anymore.

As she heated the water and pulled a tea bag out of the cupboard, she thought, *I better call my sponsor.*

Anne described to her sponsor all that had gone on, her irritation at the school, her irritation at Ken, her sudden craving. Then she found herself crying. "What's going on here?" she asked. Even as she asked the question, Anne began to identify her feelings. "I'm scared to death Ken is going to screw up big time. And I feel responsible."

"Ahh," said her friend, "so that's what's going on."

"If I'd been a different kind of mother," said Anne, "he might be a different kind of kid right now."

The language of AA helped Anne substitute a recovery behavior for her Xanax, and the language of recovery gave her enough safety and space to reflect on her feelings. She was able to take the next step and identify that she felt scared and guilty. Anne was learning something about her real self, the woman she really is. In early recovery, a woman has begun to learn the language of recovery. When she can think and she can feel, when she can know those feelings by naming them, she can begin to know who she is. She can become more than a bundle of raw nerves and instincts.

A healthy child gets support to be real. She has close, secure bonds with parents or parent figures who offer the emotional and physical attachment she needs in order to grow. She learns words to match the reality of her experiences. She learns to distinguish right from wrong, to take responsibility for her actions, and to learn about making choices. The child learns the words that will help her feel all of her emotions. Ideally, she grows up with an integration of her behavioral, cognitive, and emotional developmental tasks. This is normal child development. This is also the development you resume in recovery. Early recovery is new learning and integration of the past with the present.

Telling Her Story

With the safety of her secure attachment, her abstinent behaviors in place, and the new words she has to describe her real self, the woman begins the early recovery process of developing her "story," the narrative of who she was when she was actively addicted and out of control and of who she is now that she is sober. In AA, she learns to follow the guideline demonstrated by others: (1) tell what it was like (during active addiction), (2) tell what happened (to move her to abstinence), and (3) tell what it is like now.

As she tells the story of herself, a story that includes the reality of who she was and what she did, she comes to know herself. And with each new piece of understanding about herself, she gains confidence with which to grow, to dare to recognize another feeling that she has buried but that is a real part of who she is. Through this uncovering and opening to the feelings she has suppressed, she begins to form her own opinions and to decide what she wants. It is through this process that she becomes a richer, more multifaceted person. An authentic, unique woman. A grown-up.

Relationship with Others

There is another way that women in early recovery are similar to maturing children. They are now ready to engage the world. The infant moves from a sensing, smelling, feeding ball of instincts to a crawling, standing, walking early toddler. She gets a sure-footed sense of herself, able to cruise around from room to room, looking for Mom and Dad. She has a strong enough sense of herself that she can look outward. She wants to explore her broader world, and it is safe enough to do so now that she can stand and walk without falling all the time.

Growing up is also growing out. In new abstinence you worked to keep your focus intently on yourself. Looking outward ran the risk of pulling you back to drinking and using. Looking outward was a trigger to remind you that you were selfish for putting such a primary focus on yourself. Now it is safer to look out, to see others and to deal with others, without losing your new self.

This new mix of self and other (an "other" that is different from AA attachments) is central to early recovery. This "other" is the woman's relationship to family and friends. She's been able to form relationships with people in AA. Her abstinent behaviors are more in place, more a part of who she is. Now she's safe enough to look at the problems and adjustments that need to be made in her relationships with family and other close, personal relationships without going back to using.

This is part of the growth she needs to do in her own work. It won't happen at the beginning of her early recovery period. That's still the time for an intense focus on herself. But gradually, as she settles into the learning of this stage, including the work of the Steps, she will also begin to deal with others in a new way. Her focus on herself and her attention to others begin to operate simultaneously. Generally, part of the reason a woman uses in the first place is to avoid dealing with problems in her family, both past and present. If she is going to grow in her recovery, she has to address these difficulties. This doesn't mean yelling at family members or blaming them or giving ultimatums. It means paying attention to her own needs, listening to the needs of the "other," and working together respectfully to see how both of their needs can be met. That's a pretty picture, of course, but it doesn't often go as smoothly as that. She might find herself yelling sometimes before she remembers to calm herself and speak directly and respectfully. It's work, but work well worth doing. And fortunately, by the time she's stable in early recovery, she's solid in behavioral abstinence and is well into her inner work, so she's ready to build healthy relationships.

But remember, this focus still comes second. The woman who has recently attained a security of behavioral abstinence is still intently focused on herself and her strong attachment to AA.

Continuing to Cope with Overwhelming Emotion

Attending to real feelings and needs continues to present the woman in early recovery with intense feelings. Letting herself see her real self will bring emotion to the surface. She will need to cope with the same kind of intense feelings she was bombarded with in early transition. Facing and feeling the falseness that used to be all of her can be extremely unsettling, even traumatic. But the difference between transition and early recovery is that now she is better prepared to accept and reflect on the feelings. As the woman in recovery begins to put words to who she was and who she is, more unwelcome feelings will likely emerge. If these emotions did not arrive to overwhelm her in brand-new abstinence, they may appear now as a frightening and seemingly uncontrollable force. Much of her work involves putting words to these often still-raw feelings and integrating her past with the present.

Remember Geri, from chapter 3, who was shocked by the misery she felt when she was first sober? Who found herself feeling tormented when her husband traveled during her early recovery? When Geri had been sober for about eighteen months, she attended a meeting where a woman talked about how awful it had been for her sometimes growing up with alcoholic parents. As Geri listened, she was struck with a memory of her own behavior when she was drinking. It happened not long before she quit. Her three-year-old, Molly, got hold of some markers and brought them to her bedroom. When Geri walked in, Molly was just completing her fourth large circle in bright red on the walls that Geri had painted pale yellow six weeks earlier.

Geri lost it. She ran across the room and grabbed the marker from Molly. She started yelling, "Damn it, you little monster. You know better than to draw on the walls. What the hell's the matter with you?" She raised her hand above her head to slap the child. What Geri saw most clearly now, as she sat in her meeting, was the fear that registered in Molly's brown eyes back then. She could still see them as clearly as if it were happening now. They were wide and staring straight at her.

Geri began to sob, sitting in her metal folding chair, as she felt her daughter's panic, as she felt her own shame and sorrow at having frightened her daughter so. When she got home from the meeting, Molly was already asleep. She knelt by her bed and quietly kissed her cheek, grieving over the hurt she'd created in her little beauty's heart.

Her grief and remorse were incredibly intense. But she was able to allow herself to feel them now. She could deal with them. She knew she couldn't change that piece of the past, and Molly was too young for explanations. But she also knew she could change it going forward. That would be her way of apologizing.

Learning to Feel Good

A woman in early recovery may also have the pleasure, and surprisingly, the fear, of putting new words to positive emotion. It is quite simply true that many women are as afraid of feeling good as they are of feeling bad. They expect to feel bad, and they know how to feel bad. But they don't know how to feel good, and they're anxious about what it will mean. Many women know intuitively that they will feel guilty about feeling good—they're not supposed to be happy; they're taking something away from someone else and they should be punished.

※

Women often find themselves sabotaging any good feeling. They are afraid that feeling good will feel out of control and will therefore lead them straight back to using. Ironically, they somehow believe that feeling bad is the only way to ensure that they won't use. What a dilemma!

※

The woman in early recovery has to learn how to feel good. She has to grapple with her guilt and fear before she can tolerate such a positive experience of herself for very long. Blanca's experience illustrates this.

At nineteen years of age, Blanca had been free of drugs for almost a year. She had a big family, a close family, a family that maintained its Latino traditions and outlook. She resented the long list of rules her parents had; they simply didn't fit with the way her friends lived their lives. Her parents wanted her to come home from college every weekend. They'd fought about her living in a dorm at all, and if they called at 9:00 P.M., she'd better be in her room.

Living with these rules had been especially hard in high school. So confusing. Wanting this big lively family. Needing this family. But suffocating in it at the same time. One of the ways she fought to get her own life, to fit in with the other kids in her high school, was by using meth. It also helped give her the courage to say no to her parents. Now she was in therapy and trying to find ways to say no without hurting someone else or herself. Her therapist called it finding healthy ways to carve out a self that honored her family and herself at the same time. She wasn't sure she got the lingo, but she knew it felt good to say, "Mom, I love you, but I want to stay in the dorm this weekend and finish writing my paper on the uses of metaphor in twentieth-century Hispanic literature."

Two weekends in the last two months she had stayed on campus. She felt so grown up, so good. She planned to stay on campus one weekend next month too. It was time for her one-year medallion, and the members of her Narcotics Anonymous (NA) group said they'd take her out to celebrate.

Then she found herself dreaming. *The meth tabs were on her dresser. She took one and felt the energy rush infusing her body.* She woke up in a cold sweat from the dream, wondering what she had done. The dreams began plaguing her every night, and she woke up tired. When her mom called to tell her it was her niece's birthday and her dad would pick her up after her Friday afternoon class, Blanca could not get the word *no* out of her mouth. It was the Friday night her NA group was to take her out, but how could she let down her mom? Or her niece, for that matter? Or her aunt? Blanca just stood by the phone and cried.

Blanca, like most women in early recovery, did not realize that she was afraid of feeling good. It was particularly difficult for her, because feeling good also carried guilt about betraying her parents' values. She was growing up, but she was also growing out—out of her traditional values and into the different, more flexible mores of her college community. As she experienced the pleasure of becoming a grown-up—a separate self who could say no sometimes—the guilt set in for all the nos she was now feeling. As she experienced the quiet, everyday peace of not using methamphetemine, life was too good. She wasn't used to this feeling. She didn't know this feeling. It was strange, so strange it scared her, made her feel out of control. So she began to dream up some bad feelings. How could she feel good about herself if she wasn't being the kind of daughter a Latina is supposed to be?

You may find that, like Blanca, feeling good in recovery creates a lot of guilt and anxiety for you. Ironically, even good feelings are difficult to cope with.

Growth through Challenge: Jumping over the Hurdles

Early recovery lasts a long time. It moves along smoothly and then goes in "fits and starts," like the early days of abstinence. The woman now must deal with all the hurdles of growth, the hurdles on this road to being real. The process of settling into her recovering self can raise new flags. She experiences resistance to recovery, just like she may have felt earlier.

Resistance is a normal part of development. All growth involves fits and starts. Importantly, resistance to recovery is not necessarily a sign of relapse, though it might be. As she struggles with the anxieties and conflicts of growth, the woman may indeed relapse. A return to active addiction is always a possibility, though not always a likelihood, especially if the woman does the emotional work through the Twelve Steps.

Let's look at the hurdles.

Fear of Intimacy

The woman in recovery may struggle with her growing attachment to recovery and to anybody or anything representing recovery. She may feel intense anxiety about her needs. She has stopped drinking, and she hasn't a clue what to put in its place now that her behaviors are secure. She hears that she should still go to meetings, get a sponsor (if she doesn't have one yet), and "work the program," but she is terrified to take any steps at all.

This woman may say that she can't keep going to AA because she is a private person. She doesn't want to share. She doesn't want to need and she doesn't want to be needed by others. She wants to feel self-sufficient, the way she felt with her drug of choice. She is afraid of her dependency, and she is terrified of real human closeness and intimacy without the buffer zone created by her drugs. She is afraid she cannot hold on to who she is and be involved with another person at the same time.

Anxiety about Responsibility

The woman in recovery may want to grow and be afraid of growing at the same time because she's afraid of responsibility. She probably doesn't yet get what responsibility means. If she really knows deeply that she is responsible, she fears she will also feel guilty, full of sorrow, and ashamed. She tries to "take her own inventory," and she is suddenly talking about someone else. She can't focus on herself. There is no one there.

As Geri grew in recovery she began to understand that she needed to develop her own identity. She was talking to her sponsor about an old friend who told Geri that she should be challenging her husband about his own control issues. "Angela says the way he tries to control our kids is going to hurt them," Geri said.

"Do you see it that way?" asked her sponsor.

"Well," answered Geri, "my mom said she thinks he's overprotective."

"Is he?" asked her sponsor.

"Laura said that . . . "

Her sponsor interrupted her.

"Say 'I,'" said her sponsor. "I want to know what you think. Say 'I.'"

Geri felt like "I" was selfish and incompetent. She found it almost impossible to think about herself. Somebody else popped on her screen and out of her mouth. In the early days of recovery, it felt like there just was no Geri there.

Ongoing Shame

A woman may be struggling with inner conflict about herself and about her relationships with others. For example, she may feel torn about her identity as an alcoholic or addict. Even if she believes it absolutely, she may not like it. She may be more aware of the shame she has always associated with being out of control. Yes, she is an addict, but it hurts so much. Geri felt tremendous grief and shame about the way she had been emotionally abusive to her children when she was drinking. Fortunately, when this shame and sadness hit her at a meeting, she was able to use the understanding she had gleaned in AA to hold on to her sobriety even while she allowed herself to experience the real feelings she had about her real past.

Environmental Pulls

The woman may also be dealing with what are called "environmental pulls." This is the undertow of family, friends, and old expectations that constantly seduce her back into her old self. As we discussed in the last chapter, her family may be happy that she is in recovery, and yet they cannot understand how or what to do to support her. With luck they will quickly learn that they need to focus on themselves.

When John came home from his poker game and was greeted by Geri asking him to look at their schedules to figure out how to solve the Thursday night problem, he was annoyed. He felt like she was saying to him, "You have to change your poker night to take care of me." Right away he thought, *Yes, I do have to take care of her. If I don't, she might relapse.* But he loved his poker night. What he'd said to her before was true. He worked hard all week, and this was one of the times he could really relax and just play. He could feel the resentment starting as he answered her. "Why do I have to do all the changing so you can stay on track here? I've suffered enough already because of you." Luckily, he caught himself. "Sorry," he said. "Let's start again."

Later he lay in bed thinking about their discussion and how topsy-turvy their lives felt in spite of Geri's new sobriety. He heard an echo from the family day he'd attended during Geri's treatment. "You need to focus on yourself. Addiction is a family disease. It affects all of you. Now you need to focus on your own healing and let your partners focus on theirs." *So this is what they were talking about,* he figured. *Okay, I better check out an Al-Anon meeting.*

Family members do not always understand as readily as John did that they need to seek help for themselves. They may be unhappy and uncomfortable with the woman's new recovery because her change affects them, and they don't want to be affected. Just as she fears, her new growth and her new way of seeing herself and the world feel threatening to them.

The Twelve Step Map

Women can become thoughtful and deliberate in working the Twelve Steps as they enter early recovery. The Steps embody and outline the developmental work of recovery. They are like a map that shows you how to move forward in this journey.

You began to "work the Steps" even before you learned the language of recovery. Now, when you have the security of abstinent behaviors in place and you have begun to learn and to speak the language of recovery, you can begin to work the Steps more intentionally. Learning the language of the Steps may feel similar to the preschool and kindergarten tasks of learning the alphabet. The Steps will grow in clarity as you grow in recovery, and they will eventually become as natural to you as breathing.

Let's look briefly at how the Steps work.[1] Step One says, "We admitted we were powerless over alcohol—that our lives had become unmanageable." You started with this Step in transition. You will reach your real self when you come face-to-face with your powerlessness, when you know that powerlessness and vulnerability are the very core of who you are as a human being. Step Two says, "Came to believe that a Power greater than ourselves could restore us to sanity," and Step Three says, "Made a decision to turn our will and our lives over to the care of God *as we understood Him*." In these Steps you acknowledged your deep dependency, establishing your attachment to recovery through a new dependency relationship—the reality

---

1. This brief interpretation of the Steps is from the author's point of view. For a more detailed perspective, readers are encouraged to explore AA literature, such as the book *Twelve Steps and Twelve Traditions* (New York: Alcoholics Anonymous World Services, 1996).

of a higher power, even if this was only an idea or a possibility for you early on.

Notice here that the language of the Steps and of AA is relational. The language is the bridge that connects you with your self by establishing your connection with others. The wording of the Steps embraces a human "we" and the reality of "powerlessness." Centering the core of self in powerlessness invokes the need for a higher "other," a power greater than the self.

It is in the remaining Steps that you will build your self. You will do this by understanding and experiencing what it means to be responsible. The Fourth Step says, "Made a searching and fearless moral inventory of ourselves." In this Step, you focus on what you did. You begin to develop a self that is more than a stick figure. A self that has flesh and bones—assets and liabilities. You begin to know that you have needs and wants, some of them perfectly fine and others full of anger and resentment.

In Step Five, "Admitted to God, to ourselves, and to another human being the exact nature of our wrongs," you will reach outside of your self, outside of the isolation that kept you locked in your false self. You tell your higher power, and another person, who you are and what you did. Telling the truth will open you to have and to know your real self and to bring you into an equal relationship with all others as you vest your ultimate trust and dependence in a higher power.

In Step Six, "Were entirely ready to have God remove all these defects of character," and Step Seven, "Humbly asked Him to remove our shortcomings," you will place yourself firmly in relation to your higher power, open to seeing yourself and to change, with deference and power granted again to a higher authority. By now most women are well into a deep exploration of what this higher power meant to them in the past and what it will mean to them now. Sometimes women have great trouble establishing a deep sense of trust in "something higher." This searching and seeking will likely be central to their recovery development in the years ahead.

People in AA often say that the next five Steps are "action Steps": new behaviors, words, and feelings that will clean up the past and place you on the firm ground of your new self with new abilities and capacities to have honest, more intimate relationships with others. This comes only after you have established an honest, open relationship with your self. Again, in the AA framework, this is possible with the acceptance of your ultimate lack of power and the acknowledgment of the source of power that is outside yourself as something higher, which you will have explored and developed through the first seven Steps.

In Step Eight, "Made a list of all persons we had harmed, and became willing to make amends to them all," you accept responsibility for the harm you have done to others. The making of a list will make your agency real. You have the capacity to do damage, and you accept that you did damage, intentionally, consciously, willingly, or not.

Step Nine is a direct action Step: "Made direct amends to such people wherever possible, except when to do so would injure them or others." In this Step, you acknowledge your wrongs directly to the people you harmed, though you should be careful to determine when such open acknowledgment might do more harm than good. You should know that Steps Eight and Nine, just like all of the other Steps, are for you. You must be responsible in taking any action. These two Steps help make your past real and free you from the guilt and the burden of your wrongs. Only by acknowledging responsibility for the past and the present can anyone free themselves of the guilt of wrongdoing. Sometimes women can make restitution for harm done. Sometimes an amend can be made, but the wrong cannot be righted, and the damage cannot be undone. They must live with the past as it was and as it remains unresolved. Many women consider their right living in the present to be an amend. For instance, they cannot undo the damage they did to their children, but they can be good mothers now.

Step Ten, "Continued to take personal inventory and when we were wrong promptly admitted it," Step Eleven, "Sought through prayer and meditation to improve our conscious contact with God *as we understood Him,* praying only for knowledge of His will for us and the power to carry that out," and Step Twelve, "Having had a spiritual awakening as the result of these steps, we tried to carry this message to alcoholics, and to practice these principles in all our affairs," bring you into the present with ongoing action. These Steps are the outline for how you should live your life now. These Steps are the result of your transformation from being an active alcoholic/addict to a woman in recovery. You will pay attention to yourself every day, monitoring your behavior, thoughts, and feelings and correcting problems and missteps as soon as possible. You will stay current with honesty and acceptance of responsibility. You can do this rigorous self-assessment because you maintain a strong attachment to your higher power and continue to practice all of the Steps of your AA program. You are a woman who now knows herself in relationship—the relationship of deference to, and trust in, her higher power. This is your spiritual self. It is your relational dependence, and your deep experience of yourself as related, that gives you power now. It is a power through "other," rather than an inflated power of self.

Finally, you will work the Steps in your life. You will practice the principles. Being a woman in recovery is about all of you. It is not just "a part" of your life and your world. You will know yourself deeply and relate to others as a woman in recovery. Growing into this mature knowledge and experience of yourself will take you a long time, and it will continue to be your work for the rest of your life.

Working the Steps becomes an active process of development. You will mature into a growing and a grown-up self as you remember the past, construct your story, and acknowledge your faults and assets, past and present. Working the Steps brings you into reality, and it brings you into the present as you reflect back. The Steps are a guide to self-development. But you probably won't know this for a while. Initially, you will flounder as you hear the foreign sounds and can't make sense of them. Then these words will begin to hold you; you will feel their safety, and you will feel the relationship. You will be held by the sounds until they begin to be your own, until you begin to feel and to identify with this new language. And then these words and this language of recovery become yours.

Relapse

Just as in the transition stage, relapse is an ongoing threat in the early recovery stage as well. It's not so common now, not so much a part of the regular rhythms of the recovery process, but it does occur.

What causes a woman to go back to her active addiction now? Lots of things. She may have holes in her recovery development. Perhaps she has not learned how to be in a relationship—romantic, sexual, or friendship—without sacrificing her own desires. Perhaps she never learned how to resolve conflict without emotionally beating up the other party.

Maybe she always sees a conflict as something to be won or lost rather than resolved. A sponsor may help her go back to basics and fill in the holes. She may finally do a Fourth Step, for example, a developmental building block she always postponed. She may seek therapy to help her through this impasse. Maybe she doesn't recognize the hole and can't get moving. She is indeed stuck. Perhaps she holds on, goes around her resistance, and picks up the remedial work later.

Sometimes, she takes the drink instead. Relapse can look like the perfect painkiller for the struggles of recovery. The woman begins to doubt that she is an addict; she starts thinking that she is different from these other women, that she will be able to control her drinking. She begins to romanticize her old drinking buddies. She now can't shake her focus on the illusion of control. It temporarily eases the pain of whatever she is feeling, whatever it is that looms before her in recovery: her own feelings, the pain of her past, or the intense struggles in her relationship. All of these realities of early recovery may face her at once.

She may be struggling intensely with old feelings and old memories. The traumas of her childhood and of her adult life, including the traumas of her own active addictions, may cause her massive anxiety, depression, insomnia, and outright terror. She has flashbacks of horrific memories, or she resides in a hazy, dreamlike state of fear. It feels to her like someone is behind her; there's a reality lurking that she can't bring into focus. She strengthens her recovery behaviors and tries to work the Steps.

Hopefully, she holds on. She feels the support of others and hears how they survived the remembering. The woman in recovery strengthens her attachment to recovery people and the recovery process through the Twelve Steps, secures her recovery behaviors, and learns the new language that opens her connection to her real self.

Early recovery is a strengthening of self-development. As she settles into a positive, secure relationship with her self, a relationship she has found and grown through her dependence on recovery people and the recovery process, she moves to adult status. She is now a grown-up, a person who has a self. She has claimed agency for all that she did and for all that she does now. She accepts responsibility for herself and for no one else. She continues to learn, to accept the good and the bad, the ups and the downs, her foibles and her strengths. She is a person in ongoing recovery.

Chapter Five

Grown Up and Living Sober

THE ONGOING RECOVERY STAGE

There's no bell for this stage of recovery either. You inch your way into maturity and then, suddenly, you realize that all is well and it's been well for some time. You feel emotionally even and secure most of the time. You've been working on your development for a long time now, and all that hard work has paid off.

Being a Grown-Up

You're a grown-up and it feels good. You have a daily behavioral routine that focuses you on and in recovery, and it's natural. It feels off if you miss your routines for one day. Rarely do you need to act quickly to fend off an impulse to drink. If you do feel such a craving, you wonder what it means and where it came from, and you delve into self-exploration to find out.

The words and concepts of your Twelve Step recovery are a core part of your now-familiar self. In a sense, the Steps work you. They are automatic and feel like who you are and what you know, most of the time. You are now fluent in your language of recovery.

Your grown-up, healthy self is anchored by your awareness of your fragility, the irony of the strength in your "powerlessness." No longer do you value and long for self-sufficiency. In fact, you know that there is no such thing. You are aware of your separate self and your relational self. You exist alone and you are responsible. You also exist in relationships with others and with a power greater than yourself that you have defined and shaped as part of your development in recovery. You have been transformed, and you now live at ease and at peace—much of the time, that is.

You can still feel bad, but now you know that feeling good and feeling bad are both part of a healthy life. You deal quickly and honestly with what life brings you. Occasionally you feel downright awful, and you attend to what and why. Sometimes your dip may last a long time. There is more hard work to be done, and yes, once again, you get to do this hard work because you're in recovery. But now you know that this is normal. Life is hard. Now you have the emotional maturity to accept this reality, and you have the tools to do the work automatically.

Ongoing recovery is a filling out of recovery development. Ongoing recovery is a coming into your own that is rich; it is an expansion in the depth of your experience, your knowledge, your behavior, and your emotion. It's a bigger you, a more complex you, a grateful you.

Does this mean you've made it to the top of the long, hard climb? That you're *there*? No. By now you know that there is no "there." Ongoing recovery is not "arrival." It is recognition that development never ends. It is a time when you deepen and expand your sense of self, expand your understanding of yourself with others, and increase your capacity to live life in all its richness, both joyful and painful.

How Do I Deepen My Recovery?

Staying Open

Life will always present you with the opportunity to hurt some more, to tolerate more excavation, to experience more painful awareness, past and present. Staying open to this allows you to deepen your recovery. Of course, you don't want to go looking for pain, but when it comes, you face it and use it. You stay focused on yourself and your higher power as your source of support and your guide. You use the Steps to help you through a difficult time. You may also continue to use psychotherapy or seek this kind of help for the first time. Ongoing recovery is a time of deepening your connection with yourself, with others, and with your higher power.

As you live in recovery day after day, month after month, year after year, you uncover deep beliefs and conflicts that kept you in pain. You know that the rumble in your stomach and the sudden anxiety are alerts that something is going on deep inside. You know that it comes into focus and has meaning for you, so you don't push it away.

As an example of what I'm talking about, let's look at Carole, a woman we met in chapter 2 who was a managing editor for a national publication and who turned to Vicodin as her "stress reliever." During Carole's active addiction, her partner, Mary, left her for a while. Carole's paranoia and distortions became so intense that she almost lost her job, the job that meant so much to her. But she was lucky. The publisher recognized addiction and brought in some help. To make a long story very short, Carole went through treatment, returned to her job, and even repaired and strengthened her relationship with Mary.

It wasn't easy. Transition was horrible for Carole, and early recovery was no picnic either. She discovered fear, a blinding white fear that she would find herself alone and helpless. She relapsed several times, but she returned to recovery, stayed there, and came to love her life.

Eight years after she went through treatment she changed jobs and went to work for a women's publication. She loved it there. She could shape the attitude and content to promote her passionate commitment to opening up opportunities in the arts for all women.

Carole and Mary were considering the possibility of adopting a child when Carole found herself feeling tremendously anxious. She would awaken in the morning with a black ball in her stomach. One night she woke with a start at 3:00 A.M., shaking. In her dream she had been pouring Vicodin tablets into the palm of her hand and counting them to see how many she had left, then pouring a glass of water and gulping two of the tablets. She turned on the light and struggled to the bathroom for a real glass of water. *What is this about?* she asked herself. In the morning she said to Mary, "I'm going to call my therapist. I need a tune-up."

Progress is letting all things be, as you also learn to take action when necessary. Carole didn't pretend the anxiety didn't exist. Instead, she decided she'd get some help so she could gain a deeper understanding of herself. Progress is creating and living with a bigger space inside, a space that you now fill with new insights and feelings from the past and the present.

Letting Go of Old Defenses

Gleaning new insights and expanding your capacity to live life fully requires that you let go of some of your defenses. So what are defenses? It's a fancy way of talking about the attitudes (ways of thinking, feeling, and behaving) that protect us. Defenses are a part of human nature that help us cope with life. They can be helpful or harmful, like fire that can warm us or burn us. It depends on how we use them and how rigid they are.

Defenses help people cope emotionally, often positively. When defenses become too important and too much a part of the false self, they move from being a solution, a part of healthy coping, to the problem itself. Defenses can be used to justify or vindicate. Defenses can distort. They help an individual deny or change reality.

In active addiction, you were narrow, rigid, and highly defended. Your defenses were protecting you in some ways, but they also harmed you. You used them to get rid of bad feelings such as anxiety, anger, neediness, and self-doubt. Your defenses also kept you in your rat's cage repetition, so you kept feeling awful.

In early recovery you probably didn't recognize these defenses. Your new sense of self was still narrow, and you probably relied on old defenses to cope with the stresses of new recovery.

The old defenses get in the way of growth in ongoing recovery if they are the first place you go. They're typically slow to recede, but you are more open and flexible now and you can begin to let them go. This paves the way for you to expand your perception, thinking, and feeling. You still need some defenses, of course, as human beings always do, but they are harmful if you cannot begin to recognize them and if you rely on them to obscure reality.

Let's look at what these defenses are.

Denial

Denial is that bugaboo that haunted your active addiction days. It let you pretend to yourself that you weren't addicted. You don't need flat-out denial so much now. You can take in more and more of reality, especially your own, and you can also consider the reality of others.

Controlling Others

You don't need to immediately grasp for control of your thoughts or feelings in order to hold yourself together. And you don't need to grab for control of others either, although this issue will drive you nuts for a long time. How can you have a close relationship if you're not controlling it? It can feel dangerous. Or maybe you think you're just helping the other person because you love him or her and you know what's best. Because this is such a hard concept to grasp, let's look at an example.

Sharifa had been sober for twelve years before she truly understood how much she had been trying to control herself, her husband, Barack, and everyone around her. During the time that her addictive behaviors were active, she didn't dare talk directly with her husband about her anger or her needs. It used to be that when she would express her anger at Barack, things would get out of control, and they would both end up rageful. There were times she really thought he was going to hit her. Because of this threat of feeling out of control, Sharifa constantly tried to control conversations with Barack. The tendency to control others did not begin here. When Sharifa was young, her mother had often been rageful with her, and Sharifa had learned early in life to try to control her mother's anger by behaving and talking in certain ways.

Sharifa continued to try to exert control over others through the early years of her recovery. Barack said he didn't really get what it was that she needed from him. Besides, it seemed to her that he missed the Sharifa that was endlessly giving. He resisted going to Al-Anon or learning about the changes she was making. So Sharifa worried a lot about the gulf that was building between them, and she kept on trying to control how he responded to her.

As she went to meetings and focused on herself, she began to learn about the concept of detachment. Detachment means literally "letting go." It's a letting go of overresponsibility (having so much investment in the outcome that you have to make sure it happens in a certain way). It's a letting go of a need to control everything. Detachment is recognizing your separateness—the boundary between you and another person—and allowing this person to be responsible for him- or herself. As Sharifa and Barack went through crises in their relationship, as they fought and she worried herself sick and went to meetings and refocused on herself and what she could and couldn't change, and as she practiced living the concept of detachment, she slowly began to get it.

About eight years into Sharifa's recovery, Barack began to develop friendships with husbands of some of her friends in recovery, and he began to really understand the deep changes she had been making in her self and her life. He was behind her in recovery, but he was catching up. He slowly began to realize that he needed to focus on himself and not try to get Sharifa to change. In the last four years, they began to talk to each other at a deeper level. They talked about their individual programs. They laughed together. They expressed anger.

It was only at this point that Sharifa began to realize how much she had needed to control others. When she explained it to a woman who was younger in recovery than she was, she said: "It was so deep in me. My idea of a close relationship was to figure out how to get the other person to see or do something the way I wanted. I worked overtime to manipulate the outcome. I truly couldn't let anything unfold. I couldn't hold an open conversation because I was thinking ahead to how I wanted it to come out." Today, Sharifa and Barack can let conversations unfold without worrying about losing control. Sharifa is not so afraid of everything around her; now she can let what happens happen and know she'll be able to deal with it.

Controlling others was a terrifically hard defense for Sharifa to let go of. But as time went on and she was more and more honest with herself, she experienced something she never knew was possible. Because she was in the depths of herself with her husband, she began to feel a deeper love for him and empathy for how he felt and experienced things. And as she gained a deeper understanding for her husband that she couldn't feel before, she began to feel a deeper understanding for what her mother had experienced. She noticed that the resentment she felt toward her mother was disappearing. Slowly, her anger softened and she began to feel forgiveness. It was a feeling, not a thought or even a wish. She was able to forgive her mother, truly, deeply, honestly forgive her for her rages when Sharifa was young.

Grandiosity

You may never have felt grandiose in a way that you could recognize. You didn't feel like a big shot, and you didn't think you felt superior to others. But you did want to be able to do it all, and you thought you could. That's an inflated sense of self, no matter how bad you actually felt. Grandiosity often collapses with hitting bottom, though it may reappear throughout recovery to bolster you when you're down. Basically, grandiosity says you have no limits. By the time you reach ongoing recovery, you know you have limits, though in many instances, you don't know what they are. This is perfectly fine. You'll find out.

Projection

Projection is an old friend that tells you whatever you're feeling, thinking, or seeing belongs to someone else. Ah, how easy it used to be to see one's faults and foibles in others. Sharifa, for example, tended to project her own anger at her husband onto him. She wanted him to take her recovery seriously, to understand what she was going through and what she needed in a partner. But she didn't like to think of herself as angry. It wasn't an emotion she thought good women felt. So without realizing what she was doing, she interpreted her husband's words and actions as being angry at her, even when he wasn't. Sometimes her husband really did want her to be more attentive to him, but not as often as Sharifa thought. It was her own feeling that she wanted him to be more attentive to her that she projected onto him. You may still project your feelings onto others, but you are quick to catch yourself. You've learned to own what's yours and to believe that you're better off knowing.

Rationalization

Rationalization is making up reasons for our behavior to justify it, whether the reasons are true or not. Rationalization may remain with you as a trusted friend, though now you smile as you hear yourself explain something you're really not so sure about. Rationalization comes around whenever we think we need permission. It gives us a little more room. It usually gives an okay to something we're uncertain about. Like Sharifa, before she'd grown into forgiving her mother, saying, "I was just too busy to see my mother this month."

Expansion of Self

Your now-stable sense of security allows you to stay open, to let go of your defenses. You can question yourself more, wonder who you were, why you did what you did, and who and what you are now. You ask these questions through your Fourth Step and your Tenth Step. You ask these questions in an in-depth psychotherapy process, or you ask these questions through your religious involvement. You can tolerate asking questions and coming to know the answers. You don't need to block the answers with rigid defenses.

A New Level of Grief and Sorrow

Grief and sorrow are prominent among the feelings women experience in ongoing recovery. You probably knew these emotions during your active addiction and in your early recovery. You may have felt a terrible, inconsolable loss for your substance or for the addictive behaviors that gave you a false sense of self and connection. You may have felt sorrow and remorse for all that you did and didn't do. The pain of grief and loss may have kept you relapsing for a long time.

Now you have a different kind of grief, the grief of acceptance. It is grief for what was lost and cannot be reclaimed, a grief for what you didn't know and couldn't know. This grief comes as the pull of relapse is quiet and you no longer struggle to stay in recovery.

"Second Recovery"

Sometimes a woman reaches a point of acceptance and serenity and all goes well for many months and years, and then, one day, everything blows up. She may have a hidden trauma from the past that is now revealing itself. She may be having nightmares, and she may be suddenly anxious and doesn't know what is the matter. Naturally, but incorrectly, she asks herself, *What am I doing wrong?* In fact, she's doing right. She now has the internal strength and the support of her program and her relationship with her higher power to tolerate painful uncovering work.

Some people call this a "second recovery," in the sense that the woman gets to go digging once again. She gets to feel out of control, scared, and ignorant about what's happening. Many feel like they're starting over again. But not so. This is another deepening of self and more recovery work. Now the woman can tolerate feeling out of control and staying with the emotion to see where it leads. She stays close to her Twelve Step program to be sure her abstinence is secure while she tackles the hard emotional work.

I've talked in earlier chapters about how memories or feelings about past trauma rise to the surface during transition and early recovery. You'll recall that this experience of trauma is overwhelming, a feeling of utter helplessness, a dying of the self. You'll recall, too, that these memories and feelings are often relapse triggers and that a woman experiencing these probably needs professional help.

These memories or feelings may continue to bubble to the surface during ongoing recovery or may even appear for the first time later in recovery. A woman may now remember physical, sexual, or emotional abuse that was a onetime horror or an ongoing part of her "normal" life. She may have grown up with an alcoholic father or mother, or both, a mentally ill parent or sibling, or a chronically ill and always-on-the-verge-of dying parent. There are lots of kinds of trauma and many of them seem perfectly normal to the people who are living with them. But they create an unsafe family environment and an unsafe sense of self. Trauma involves a feeling of impending threat or doom. A feeling that something is wrong or something is going to be wrong, terribly wrong. And indeed, something is wrong.

As Carole considered adopting a child with Mary, it reawakened her own childhood fears of helplessness and abandonment. Her parents were both high-achieving, driven alcoholics. Now in therapy again, Carole remembered the thundering fights her parents had when they were drunk. She remembered the butcher knife sailing past her father's head and sticking into the wall. She remembered her dad's fist connecting with her mother's jaw. The images made her stomach roil. She remembered how her parents had jointly turned their fury on her when she showed them a note from a teacher saying she was getting her assignments in late. Her mother's hand had felt like a switch when it connected with Carole's cheek.

These weren't new images. They weren't new memories. But as she connected them with her own anxiety about raising a child, she began to realize how deep her fear went, how worried she was that she couldn't do a good job of being a parent. Her childhood fear that she would be abandoned if she didn't perform well was coming up to haunt her again.

Along with therapy, Carole added an extra meeting and talked to her sponsor daily for a while. She needed the extra support. Carole was able to face her pain immediately in ongoing recovery. Instead of running from it, she used it to deepen her understanding of who she was and what she needed. She had developed a secure reliance on a solid program to help her through emotional turmoil or even meltdown.

Who Am I Now?

To review here, as you continue to open yourself to all of your experience, rather than shutting it down and out of your consciousness, you glean a stronger and larger sense of who you are. You get to have new beliefs and new ways of relating to others. You are flexible, open to questioning yourself, and open to new insight. You experience your dependence and your separateness, and you know the difference between unhealthy and healthy detachment and disengagement. You know the difference between detaching with love that is a real letting go, that gives you a real separation, and detaching with anger or desperate need that keeps you tightly bound together.

You also have a bigger capacity for feeling. Now you know what acceptance means and what it feels like. You know forgiveness that emerges at a deep level from within. You cannot will yourself to think or feel a different way. But you will be able to think and feel differently as you gain a deeper sense of yourself. You have a capacity to understand yourself and others at a deep level, to be accepting, and to forgive.

Expansion of Self and Other

In ongoing recovery you get to establish and build new, closer, richer, and more intimate relationships with others. This kind of intimacy is a core of healthy sobriety.

It is not an intimacy you need to make you whole. You are already whole, and it is your whole self that you now bring to relationships with others. You will find out what it means to be independent, to be interdependent, and to really feel a healthy kind of dependence. You can do all this now because you can tolerate the vulnerability that comes with being real, with being responsible, and with being a grown-up. But it's not easy, nor smooth, as Geri discovered.

After eleven years of sobriety, Geri enjoyed watching her daughter, Molly, make forays into quasi-romantic territory. It was fun seeing the pride in her son, Willy, when he cooked occasional dinners for the family. Geri and John and the two kids ate dinner together at least four nights a week, and they had great discussions—sometimes fights too. The family knew how to have fun together and how to argue, and cry, and come back together again.

Geri, John, and their two children lived with a deepening sense of new intimacy. But now she was faced with conflict: She had more individual work to do, and she feared that doing the work would interfere with her family's comfort and stability. Geri was beginning to realize how terrified she had been as a youngster of her mother's iron fist. Geri needed to deepen her relationship with herself by remembering the past, but she knew this work would take time from her family.

And she worried: Would she find herself crying a lot? Would she get short with John and the kids as she did this work? Would they be mad at her? Would they hang in there with her? This dilemma is a core of building and maintaining intimate relationships: How do I hold on to myself, keep growing, and stay close and connected with others? How do I do my own work when it threatens others? When do I hold on to my view and live with conflict, when and how do I compromise without losing myself, and how do I live with others not coming to see things my way? This was the same dilemma Sharifa was facing when she feared that her husband would never do the work he needed to do.

There are no easy answers to these questions. Nor are they ever answered once and for all. These dilemmas are the stuff of living. You solve one conflict and there's another one, next in line. Every conflict is different and needs to be resolved differently. You yielded on the last, and this time you hold firm. How do you tolerate this kind of fluidity and absence of absolutes—no always-binding rules (except don't drink or use) and no "fixes"?

It takes a lot of trust, because you are not going to accomplish these challenges by trying to control it all or by waiting to move until your partner says it's okay. Sharifa had to take the plunge. So did Geri. She had to do the work, and she had to let her family be. They got it eventually.

Some family members lead the way in "getting it," some follow later, and some never understand. Being a healthy woman in recovery means you are committed to being honest, to seeing and feeling, regardless of what others think, do, or feel. You may think that this commitment to yourself will guarantee downfall—that you'll lose everyone and everything. But being committed to your own growth does not mean a loss of all others. It does mean that you won't be able to guarantee a happy-ever-after kind of agreement and sameness with those you love. Instead, you come to see that you can think, feel, and see things differently than the person you love. Or that your growing differences will mean a parting of your ways. You just can't know before you see and feel and know what is real.

Deepening your relationship with yourself and with others keeps you feeling vulnerable. This gives you an opportunity for new closeness with others. It's scary and good at the same time. This is the opposite of what you always dreamed self-esteem would be. You thought you needed to feel powerful, to feel grand, to be the mistress of your world. You thought you should never feel anxious or alone. But now you feel all of these and you feel at peace.

Relapse

Most women in ongoing recovery do not relapse, though they may feel unsure of themselves and the solidity of their recovery at times. They may wonder, just like they did early on, if the feelings they are having are a warning of relapse or a part of normal growth. Now they know how to find out. They continue to work their recovery programs and let the process work for them. This is a combination of taking action—recovery action—and letting go, of working the program and paying attention to the inner self, of listening and allowing space to hear.

Sometimes women will develop other addictive behaviors during recovery—they turn to food suddenly after many years of recovery from alcohol or other drugs. Or they realize that they're revved up, thinking compulsively about shopping or the fun they had at a gambling casino. The woman with a solid recovery will pay attention. She'll register the change in her feeling and behavior, and hopefully, she'll seek help if she begins to lose her focus on recovery.

This kind of revving up, or sudden feeling of intense need, used to bring an instant, impulsive action. She would drink, pop a pill, eat, or head to the gambling table. Not anymore. Now she can tolerate registering and holding the feeling, while seeking healthy support. Then she looks at what it all means. This is healthy recovery.

PART THREE

The Paradoxes of Recovery

In this section, we'll explore the major elements of change that women experience in recovery. At the heart of each of these elements lies paradox, a concept that's been mentioned repeatedly in this book. The dictionary says a paradox is a statement that seems opposed to common sense, yet is true; something with seemingly contradictory qualities In short, a paradox is *not what you think it is*. At first blush it doesn't make logical sense; it feels mysterious. But when you look more deeply, it's true.

Paradox involves surprise. Paradox is all about surprise in logic and meaning. The surprise, the incongruity, that greets us in paradox is similar to the mechanisms of humor. The surprise of an incongruous pairing is what makes something funny. We laugh at the incongruity, the connection of opposites and contradictory premises. The punch line catches us off guard, and we suddenly see something we couldn't see or predict as we followed logically. But here comes the surprise, and it catches us on another level of meaning. With humor, basic premises are altered so you have the shock of the punch line. Or you experience the shock of the impossible, as in the injunction: "Be spontaneous!"

The change in logical premise that makes something funny is

similar to the change in meaning that occurs when people move from active addiction to recovery. Coming into recovery involves shock, the surprise of a fundamental change in premise and a fundamental change in meaning. It's the shock of the "aha," the sudden illumination that occurs when a puzzle finally makes sense and you can't believe you couldn't see it before. A woman will shift from believing, "I am not an alcoholic; I can control my drinking," to seeing and believing deeply, "I am an alcoholic; I have lost control." And she doesn't know exactly how she made the change. It may come as a sudden leap, a shock, or it may come slowly, methodically, as she hunts for the puzzle pieces and finally finds the one that brings everything into focus. Now she sees. In this process of radical change she doesn't get new glasses; she gets new eyes.

Many women in recovery describe the radical changes they've experienced as conversion. More than a century ago, philosopher William James described religious and psychological conversion as paradoxical: "A self hitherto divided becomes unified."[1] But how conversion occurs is mysterious, and the process of getting there is unexpected and often makes no sense. Women in recovery have gone from internal war to feeling whole, but they often don't know how they got there.

This is why paradox is so central to the radical changes a woman experiences in recovery. Recovery involves transformation, a kind of change so radical there is no continuity and no clear way of knowing how you got there. Philosopher Thomas Kuhn put it well in describing the nature of scientific revolutions: "What were ducks before are rabbits afterward."[2] Women just aren't the same as they were before.

Recovery is a turnaround in everything: new attachment, identity, belief, behavior, and emotion. But it's not going from bad ducks to good ducks. You're going from ducks to rabbits, from false to real.

1. William James, *The Varieties of Religious Experience: A Study in Human Nature* (Cambridge, Mass.: Harvard University Press, 1903).
2. Thomas Kuhn, *The Structure of Scientific Revolutions* (Chicago: University of Chicago Press, 1962), 111.

In this section, we'll look at the key paradoxes of addiction and recovery, why they're so difficult to grasp, and why it's essential to come to terms with the notion, "It's not what you think it is." We will explore four paradoxes: (1) the power in powerlessness, (2) the wholeness of a divided self, (3) independence built on dependence, and (4) relying on others although you're responsible for yourself (the apprentice model of learning in AA).

Chapter Six

The Power in Powerlessness

"Oh no," you say. "I hate this. Not more about being powerless. Do I have to feel and remember how out of control I was? Do I have to feel and remember that I am still basically and fundamentally out of control?" If you are well along in recovery, you say this tongue in cheek because you know your new self is built on the foundation of powerlessness. This is the number one paradox in recovery: The cornerstone of your strength is your acceptance that you are powerless

When you begin recovery, you recognize and accept that you have lost control. Powerlessness is the loss of ability to know when to stop, to be able to stop, and even to want to stop whatever is driving you. It might be drinking, using other drugs, eating, gambling, spending, having sex, smoking, or experiencing out-of-control attachment to and behavior with another person (codependency). Whatever its form, being powerless is being out of control. It's being the victim of your own obsessions and compulsions to repeat; once again, to do it when you don't want to do it. Or to do it when you do want to and the hell with the consequences.

An Itch That Won't Go Away

When you're in the throes of active addiction, you know deep down that you're powerless, and this knowledge is agonizing. Still, the "merry-go-round" of being out of control and denying it at the same time catches you in its grip. This is how Geri explained her experience:

> I cringed every time I heard the word *powerless*. I had a *problem* with alcohol and that's the only way I could think about it. I wasn't powerless over my drinking or anything else. I just overdid it a bit now and then. At first it drove me crazy to hear people in AA go on and on about their great discovery—that being powerless had set them free. Not me. I wasn't going there. It took me years before I really got it.

Substituting Addictions

You'll likely get lots of chances to see that you're powerless, just like Geri. That's because really and truly accepting that you are powerless about everything, not just drinking, takes time. It's an understanding you gain only through repeated experiences. Many women substitute new unhealthy dependencies for the old substance or behavior, remaining actively addicted to something or someone well into recovery.

You may remember that Geri went for the ice-cream bowl to try to calm herself when she first entered the shock of recovery. It was an old coping behavior, something she had used to stuff her feelings before she started to rely on alcohol. As she grew out of her clothes, she realized she was substituting food for drink, and then she turned to shopping. And once again, she recognized her powerlessness. Only after six years of recovery did Geri really get it. Let's listen to Geri again.

> Sometimes I think of myself as a creature of control. I give up control of one thing, accept that I'm powerless, and in an instant I'm on to controlling something else. You'd think I'd get it, and I do, actually. But that need for control is like an itch. There it is again.

Women and Powerlessness

Even though powerlessness is fundamental to being human, women have a particularly difficult time coming to terms with this reality. There have always been, and still are, countless personal, social, cultural, and political barriers that hamper a woman's ability to really feel and accept her powerlessness.

One of these is the pressure on women, historically, and even still today, to be "good." Until recently, it was believed that only certain kinds of women—promiscuous women—could be so fallen as to be labeled addicted. Women were idealized as virtuous, selfless caretakers who could not lose control. When a virtuous woman lost control to an addiction, it was disguised as medication, something to calm her nerves. Of course, the reality was that her hidden addiction was visible to all—a woman with a well-known secret. But it was still clothed in respectability.

This terrible double bind of secret need and invisibility was created by the morality of early gender views. Being openly addicted and out of control was viewed as masculine, a symbol of male character and male privilege. It was also often an expression of male dominance. Women were viewed as morally flawed if they openly had needs or wishes to drink. Women felt invisible and needed to behave as if they were. Yet women had needs, and they did exist. Secret nipping or popping tranquilizers became the only means of living out this double standard and double life.

The fight for feminist equality, as important as it was, brought along with it a pressure that made it hard for women to accept their powerlessness. A woman's right to drink, to use other drugs, to gamble, to smoke, and to spend became linked with a social-political struggle that focused on an external enemy: those men and women who would deny equality to women. This political focus mobilized women in a war against the dominant males. Women were used to directing their attention outside of themselves in their role as caretaker, so adding an enemy simply reinforced their external focus. But women also need to turn inward. They need to see that the battle with addiction is inside.

Again, as important as it was, this drive for equality through social and political empowerment also paradoxically created internal difficulties for women. This kind of drive for power, so characteristic of the political world, tends to reinforce a woman's downward, repetitive struggle with addiction. The focus on gaining power can work against a woman's capacity to see herself as powerless. It can even work against her ability to see herself at all. That's what happened to Carole, who came of age just as the feminist movement was really gaining steam. As she told her story at a meeting, she said:

I joined the feminist movement with great excitement. I declared myself equal and easily got into the gender war. Men were to blame, and it was our job to fight them and the patriarchy that kept them in power. This was a good war, and we won a lot. But I was riding the crest of my political anger with nightly drinking and pot smoking. It all felt so liberating. I could fight for my rights and I could drink and smoke all I wanted. You couldn't have said the word *powerless* to me back then. I was full of power, though I was also completely out of control.

An Inside War

According to anthropologist Gregory Bateson, addiction is always about the self. It is always, ultimately, an individual issue. Of course, others may be involved. But, ultimately, coming to terms with your addiction is coming to terms with the "self" and the self alone. Being addicted is an inside war. One part of a woman believes she can control her drinking while another part is victim to her loss of control. She determines she will win this inside war and then watches herself lose, over and over again.

When she hears that she should fight for power over others, she applies that to herself. She strengthens her belief in the power of control. She should be able to control herself, and she will work harder to achieve it. Sadly, she intensifies her denial and defensiveness. She works harder to maintain her belief in her own power. Carole continued in her story:

I was so full of myself. When I had those little doubts, that voice inside that said, "You're drinking too much," I'd square my shoulders and tell that voice to hush up. I was strong and I could take control and stay in control. Then when I reduced the drinking, I started on pills.

The language of the gender wars is aggressive. It's a striving for "power over." It's a win "against." In contrast, the language of recovery is accepting, which paradoxically sets the groundwork for transformational change. A woman gives up trying to achieve "power over" and instead accepts her lack of power and her need for help. In recovery, loss of control is not equated with failure. On the contrary, as a woman accepts responsibility for herself, she gains a different kind of power, a power that comes from within.

Trauma and Powerlessness

Another pressure that makes it particularly difficult for women to recognize and accept their powerlessness is the experience of trauma. We've looked at the effect of trauma several times so far. Now it comes up again.

Women have experienced all kinds of trauma at the hands of others, both as adults and while growing up. How difficult for a woman to come to terms with being powerless over her ability to control herself, when being tragically, helplessly powerless was her common experience as a child. She may have grown up living with chronic abuse, living with others who repeatedly lost control of themselves. Or she may have been abused repeatedly as an adult by a powerful partner. This woman may have worked hard to make sure she would never feel so vulnerable, that she would never again experience herself as helpless.

For many of these women, becoming addicted was the solution to feeling helpless, the answer to finally getting control. They learned that, with the help of their addiction, they could shut themselves down or open up at will. They could have what they wanted, and they could quiet the pain. They could release feeling or make it go away.

Mai Lee, who, you will remember, was sexually abused by her uncle before she even entered high school, struggled with the idea of powerlessness as she quit drinking. Shortly after her uncle moved out of her family's home, she decided that she would never trust anyone and would never be dependent on anyone for anything. She explained to the women in her new AA meeting at college: "People had hurt me too much. I had decided I would depend on myself. I've lived with this 'truth' ever since, and it's incredibly hard to let it go. I depended on myself and never needed anyone, and I did it by being addicted."

What a tragic, though understandable, decision she made. She treated one difficulty by creating another. She became the creator of her own trauma of powerlessness and loss of control. With her addiction, she became the perpetrator and the victim. A woman in this position might have other victims too, which is a horrible reality to face.

⚜

The woman who has experienced trauma adds extra resistance to feeling and recognizing that she is powerless. Being powerless reminds her too soon and too intensely of her childhood. Being powerless reminds her that she was victimized, she lived with horror, and then she did it too. It's a lot to grasp early on. So she struggles against this understanding.

⚜

It's important for women to have help in dealing with their own loss of control and to have help in dealing with the traumatic powerlessness they have also experienced with others. Accepting the reality of powerlessness is the first step toward healing. Learning to live with the ongoing truth of powerlessness is the work of recovery.

The Power in Powerlessness

The idea of being powerless, of being out of control, is even harder to understand than it might seem. It is very difficult to come to terms with the concept and the reality of being powerless. It's especially hard for women who have a long history of being victimized or repressed by people who do have power, both on a socio-political level and on a personal level. This experience of being hurt by their powerlessness has made it even more difficult for women who are addicted to admit their powerlessness over their addictions.

For all the women I've talked about so far in this book, really "getting" the fact that they were powerless seemed to take forever. It took years and multiple attempts at gaining control before they realized they just couldn't do it. As we've seen, many women in recovery substitute one addiction for another as they desperately try to hold on to some modicum of control. Being powerless is anathema; it means second-class citizenship and misery.

This is where the paradox comes in. When it comes to addiction, admitting you are powerless means freedom. When women finally, deeply realize that they are powerless over their addictions, when they accept it and quit fighting it, they feel a great sense of freedom. They are finally free of the constant, exhausting, and inevitably defeating effort to try to get control, both of themselves and others. They get the freedom to quit trying to manipulate the people around them, to control their environment. If they can't possibly control, then they are free to rely on someone or something else for help. They don't have to be perfect anymore.

Even more important, they get the gift of themselves. As they accept responsibility for getting to a place where they were powerless over their addiction, they get to know and nurture a real self. They get the freedom to be who they really are: someone who is complex, less than perfect, sometimes good or kind or loving or competent and sometimes not.

For a woman in recovery, acknowledging and accepting her powerlessness gives rise to a different kind of power as well as freedom. This power is about capacity, having the capacity to know yourself, to be honest with yourself and with others, to grow. It is about the ability to act, to do things you want to do.

Central to the power and freedom in powerlessness is a deep acceptance of limits. A woman knows that as a human being, she can't do it all and she isn't all. She knows that being powerless means she must constantly pay attention to what she can do and what she can't. What she can control and what she can't. What she is responsible for and what she's not. What kind of power she has and doesn't have. This is what that phrase "the wisdom to know the difference" in the Serenity Prayer is all about.

❖

The Serenity Prayer, "God grant me the serenity to accept the things I cannot change, the courage to change the things I can, and the wisdom to know the difference," credited to theologian

Reinhold Neibuhr, has been a central element of treatment and recovery groups for decades.

⚜

As you begin to live with a foundation of powerlessness and learn what your limits are, you will also discover the power of boundaries.

A boundary is the place where you end and another person begins. It is the separate "you." It is what allows you to say yes and no. Becoming sober is the first yes, the first declaration of a new self. Becoming sober is also the first limit and the first boundary. A woman sets the limit of no alcohol and she sets the boundary of her separate self as she declares, "I am an alcoholic." "I have lost control" is an acceptance of personal responsibility—also a boundary between herself and all others. Boundaries are what you develop as you learn who you are and assert yourself. Boundaries give you the capacity—the power—to live as an active, responsible agent on your own behalf.

It takes a long time to develop healthy boundaries and healthy dependencies and to alter addictive behavior. So you may find that you're face-to-face with feeling and being powerless long after you've put down the drink, the needle, the pill, or the pastry. The challenge for the woman in recovery is how to maintain a deep belief in the reality of her powerlessness, how to see the power in powerlessness, and how to apply it to the rest of her life. No matter how long a woman has been in recovery, she will never be without opportunities to feel powerless and, if she's lucky, to recognize her liberation, her equality, and her security in this truth.

Chapter Seven

The Wholeness of a Divided Self

ACCEPTING CONFLICT

What is conflict and why is it so important to understanding the hard road of recovery? It's important because avoiding conflict has sent women toward addiction and kept women from recovering. I'm not talking about the kind of conflict where you try to beat somebody or win a battle with another person, though that kind of conflict can do damage. I'm talking about internal conflict, the battle of opposing forces inside the self. I'm also talking about the kind of conflict you face in relationships when you're trying to do what's best for all of you but it just doesn't work.

These kinds of conflicts are uncomfortable, even painful and miserable. Nevertheless, it is a discomfort we all have to live with because it's a normal part of life. As you get to know the real you—and remember, getting to know the real you is the primary work of recovery—you feel all kinds of conflict. Conflict about "bad" traits, conflict about negative feelings, conflict about your strengths and your good feelings, conflict about choices. The first impulse is often to try to get control of that uncomfortable feeling, to get rid of that conflict. But this kind of control is part of what got you in trouble in the first place.

Like the paradox that we explored in chapter 6, the second paradox I want to explore with you also has to do with powerlessness and with giving up the need to control. But in this instance, it's about giving up trying to control your internal life, the uncomfortable feelings of conflict. Conflict, both internal and within relationships, may be uncomfortable, but it's also the stuff of life. To ignore it, deny it, or try to escape it is to escape part of life. You end up allowing only a portion of your self to live. A false self. Not the real you. You can't be a healthy, mature, whole person unless you also can accept conflict, because conflict is part of life. This brings us face-to-face with the second paradox: The path to wholeness is acceptance of a divided, conflicted self.

Conflict Is Normal

Internal Conflict

Philosophers have long pondered the concept of conflict. The early Greek philosopher Heraclitus identified internal conflict as a divided self, a state of being that is central to human nature. In the nineteenth century, Georg Wilhelm Friedrich Hegel suggested that a polarity of opposites exists as a force of natural development. He believed in the "unity or identity of opposites." The point I want to make here is that both of these philosophers—as well as people today—agree that having a divided self is natural. Internal conflict is a normal state of being. To feel *this* way, but on the other hand, think *that* way. To think *this,* but on the other hand, think virtually the *opposite.* Another word you will often hear used to refer to this divided state of being is *ambivalence.*

Conscious and Unconscious Divisions

Internal conflict can be both conscious and unconscious. Unconscious conflict is the difference between what you consciously see and believe to be true and what you know deep down, at a subconscious or unconscious level, is true. It's outside of your awareness when it's unconscious. Conscious conflict, on the other hand, involves feelings you are aware of as you struggle with opposing beliefs, wishes, or motives, with conflicts you recognize. You want to be the winner, and you're afraid of winning, so you tell yourself that you don't care. You believe that you only want the best for your friends, and you resent their good fortune at the same time. You want your own life, and you feel guilty for wanting it. On and on it goes.

Conflict in Relationships

Conflict is also a normal part of relationships. It occurs when individuals have desires and opinions that clash. This, of course, is inevitable. It doesn't matter how much two individuals care about each other; because they are separate selves, they will find that sometimes they are on opposite sides of a question. Relationship conflicts might be small, like whether dinner is best eaten at 6:00 P.M. or 8:00 P.M., or whether you like a particular movie or not. But sometimes conflicts are more significant, such as where to live or how to raise kids, or what you need and want and feel you're not getting. When this occurs with a person you care about, conflict in the relationship becomes internal conflict as well. It creates conflicted feelings about how to be true to yourself and how to fulfill your responsibilities in your relationship. How can both be in good shape at the same time?

The conflict that exists in relationships tends to be felt

acutely by women. Not only are women raised to put them-selves behind others, but they tend to look at the world, to understand the world, in the context of relationships. And so when a relationship is presenting difficulty, it can be very hard for a woman to figure out how to balance the needs of the relationship and her own separate, personal needs. A woman in recovery will struggle intensely with this conflict: Who or what is first? But once again, this makes it harder to accept that conflicted feelings about a friendship, a marriage, a partnership, even a parent-child relationship, are perfectly normal.

Internal conflict is both normal and uncomfortable. Some-times it's so uncomfortable that it's painful, even excruciating, and we want to leave it behind. This is understandable, but it doesn't serve us well. When we try to escape the pain of am-bivalence, to deny that we have any internal conflict, we get in trouble. In fact, most theorists see that addiction starts as a solution to some kind of problem or dilemma. Addiction seems to quiet what can't be resolved, but only temporarily, of course. Soon it makes the conflict worse.

Conflict and Women

Between the Ideal and the Real

Conflict for women goes way back. Society has set strict roles for women, roles that are set like bars in a cage around who they can be. While big changes have occurred during the last four decades, there is still a lot of pressure on women to live out certain roles. They are supposed to be loving and kind and sweet and giving. They are supposed to be deferential and passive and demure. Women are not supposed to have needs, wishes, or motives. Women are not supposed to exist, really, except to care for others.

It's hard to know the real you when there is so much of you that's not supposed to exist. But the fact is that every woman has multiple parts—various needs, wishes, motives—and she often holds them in secret, from others as well as from herself. As a woman in recovery begins to know the real self, the parts she wasn't supposed to have, she feels conflict. A woman can end up feeling conflict about virtually anything.

Fear of Negative Traits and Feelings

As you grow in recovery, you become aware of things about yourself that you'd perhaps rather not know. Things like the fact that you have a nasty side to yourself. Selfishness. Greed. Envy. Anger. Hate. Never mind that these traits are normal and every human being has them. You'd rather not. You feel lousy about them. You feel especially lousy about them because you're a woman. A good woman isn't supposed to have these nasty traits. So it's a double whammy. These are things that come with being alive, and many people don't celebrate these parts of themselves, but there's still less room for women to be angry and aggressive and selfish than there is for men. You try hard to get rid of these traits, these feelings, but you can't, and you feel conflicted. Or you try hard to pretend you don't have them, and you feel conflicted.

❧

Many women confuse internal conflict with character defects, and they struggle in recovery to grasp the difference. Like conflict, character defects are normal and part of being human.

❧

Character traits are the qualities of a personality, the ingredients of a self: who we are, what we feel, and what we value and believe in. Character traits may also be character defects when the trait habitually gets in the way of healthy growth. For example, say a woman has a character trait of using anger as a defense. She may intensify this character trait if she cannot recognize or accept that she feels conflicted. She may believe that she shouldn't feel any bad feelings, so she works hard to deny the reality that she does feel negatively. She may act out her "character defects" with herself and with others in an attempt to quiet or resolve her conflicts. So both the anger and the conflicts get worse. More intense, more unresolvable.

This can get confusing. A woman may very well recognize that she feels conflict, but she decides that the conflict she feels is itself a character defect, something she should work to eliminate. Instead of being able to accept the complexity within herself, she works harder to make the bad go away.

Remember the paradox? The path to wholeness is through accepting the divided parts of the self. Part of that is accepting that the negative parts of the self exist. Let's look at the example of Tenaya.

When Tenaya was growing up, her sister was chronically ill and spent a lot of time at home. Tenaya thought the only way she could be a good person was if she stayed home with her sister and kept her company. This caused Tenaya to miss out on a lot of activities, and she didn't have many friends. She was angry about this, but she also felt guilty. She didn't feel like she could be a good person and be angry, so both the guilt and the anger remained subconscious.

At fourteen years old, Tenaya joined a gang. She still hadn't yet realized her feelings of anger and guilt; she just knew she wanted to have fun and to have friends. Getting high helped her escape the guilt she felt about having friends. For a while, it was heaven. She did everything: alcohol, other drugs, pills, anything she could eat or swallow or shoot. But ultimately, she realized that she felt alone; all she had were her drugs and her longing.

When Tenaya went into treatment, she still felt the anger that she had felt growing up and the guilt for having friends, but she still didn't know it. She wanted to make friends in treatment, but she gave off vibes that said, "Get away from me!" One night she brought it up in her treatment group. "This isn't a very friendly group," she complained. "I'm trying very hard to make friends, but it feels like no one here likes me much."

A woman sitting next to her in the circle challenged her. "I do like you," she said, "but it seems like every time I get involved in a conversation with you, you hit me with a sarcastic remark. I end up feeling like you don't think much of me."

A woman across the room chimed in. "I was going to come talk to you tonight before the meeting began, and as I started toward you, you turned your head in the other direction. I got the distinct impression you didn't want to talk to me."

Tenaya was startled. She didn't realize that she was pushing people away because she was still busy denying she had any anger. She still disapproved too much of that part of herself to let herself see it. She didn't want to feel angry, but she couldn't get over it when she didn't even know she was feeling it. So she kept on feeling rejected instead.

When she had been in recovery for six years, she began to understand the internal conflict she was experiencing. She was doing her usual Tenth Step work, and she thought about a conversation she'd had earlier in the day. As she replayed it in her mind, she realized something. She remembered throwing a sarcastic remark at the woman and seeing her face freeze for a moment. Suddenly she was able to tune into the anger that prompted her remark, even though it wasn't anger at the woman herself. She said, "I just saw it. I was the one doing the rejecting. I pushed away and I felt rejected." Suddenly it was clear to her that she had always felt conflict.

It was a powerful moment for her. Tenaya had always struggled with internal conflict during her recovery: She wanted to be sober and she wanted to belong in AA, but she kept rejecting any feeling of belonging. One day she saw what had been subconscious: Belonging meant she'd left her sister behind. As long as she didn't feel that she belonged anywhere outside of her family when she was growing up, she could cope with her guilt. She didn't have to face the anger that lay under her guilt. Now, feeling a part of AA triggered this same old guilt and anger. Eventually, she was able to more clearly separate the past from the present and enjoy a feeling of belonging in AA.

Fear of Inner Strength

Ironically, women can feel even more conflicted about their strengths than their weaknesses. Far more so, in fact. They can feel more troubled about the strong and positive parts of themselves than the negative and weak parts of themselves. Women have powerful feelings and desires and opinions. They can be daring and assertive, sometimes on behalf of others, but also on behalf of themselves. However, this way of being in the world is outside of the traditional roles women have occupied. So it causes them conflict when they act on their desires or opinions. It even causes them conflict when they realize they have these desires and opinions. They believe that they shouldn't have wants and needs, so the fact that they do causes them anxiety.

What if a woman acts on the basis of her inner strength? Say she speaks her mind. She may end up feeling guilty that she upstaged someone. She may end up worrying that she offended someone or that she won't be liked. Women fear the power they really do have, the power of having feelings and desires and opinions, of having a self and acting on it.

Remember Carole, the editor whose high-achieving parents were both alcoholics? Carole was used to being a strong woman. She had excelled in her job in publishing, climbing to the top very quickly. She was proud of what she had accomplished. And despite the fact that she resented co-workers when she imagined they were trying to get her job, she also worried that she had offended people when she spoke out in meetings. She worried about offending the staff she supervised when she gave them difficult but important feedback. She worried about people thinking she was a difficult woman, or an arrogant woman, or a selfish woman. In recovery she began to realize that she had mixed feelings about her success.

But she really thought she had put that all behind her by the time she was fourteen years into her recovery. By then she and Mary had adopted Kim, a little girl from Korea. When Kim started preschool, there were very few children of Korean ancestry around and no cultural services. Carole began to campaign to bring more cultural awareness into the schools. And even as her campaign was gaining momentum and she was getting calls from other parents offering help, she started to feel tremendously anxious. Once again, she found herself haunted by worries that she was offending people, that they would think her arrogant. She was a strong and powerful woman, yet she still worried that these parts of herself should not exist.

It's All My Fault

Coping with internal conflict is complicated by the fact that, for many women, it is second nature to assume that everything is their fault, to accept blame automatically for any reality that doesn't match the ideal. And it's also second nature to assume that women want the best for themselves and others and will behave accordingly to achieve this same ideal. So when they fail, the guilt is severe. Women believe that they should make everyone happy, fix all that is wrong, and never have needs of their own in the mix. They should be paragons of virtue.

❖

Drinking and using give many women the illusion that they can control the imperfections, the flaws that mar the ideal. Turning to something—alcohol, food, sex, shopping—gives women a "time-out," a space of their own that is not focused on others. Pausing to nip, to shoot, to swallow that pill, gives women a breather. It's a way to take care of themselves without appearing to neglect others.

❖

That's how it started for Geri. With her two young children and her husband, she just kept going, never stopping all day long. Late at night, after she got the kids to bed, she'd go to her hideaway and sit with her brandy. She could finally slow down and get a feeling for herself. This was precious time. As we know, Geri ended up in trouble because she couldn't stop. One brandy became two and then three. She'd wake up at 5:00 A.M. with an empty bottle. In recovery, she learned to claim time for herself. It was essential, but it was so hard to do. She felt guilty about needing her own space.

For Geri and many others, addiction is fuel. It helps them maintain their stamina and gives a false sense of strength. Indeed, the substance or behavior is a woman's best friend. She can believe she really is a superwoman, until she starts to crack. And then she has to face the fact that she has needs and the conflicted feelings she has about that.

Conflict and Recovery

To review here, most women don't know conflict is normal and work hard to make it go away. Conflict causes pain. A woman creates a false self as she denies that conflict exists, and this creates more pain. It's a painful compromise that stunts her growth. Using alcohol or other drugs quiets the conflict and pain. And then makes it worse. Eating or drinking or shopping makes the bad feelings go away, and then causes other bad feelings. It becomes a vicious cycle: The woman believes that she should not feel conflict, that she should be clear about everything, and that having negative as well as positive feelings, having mixed feelings, having ambivalence, are all signs of failure or poor character.

Letting Go of Control

As we've seen, many women confuse internal conflict with character defects, and they struggle in recovery to grasp the difference. They think that being conflicted is itself a character defect, something to be eradicated with healthy recovery.

They believe that they are not supposed to feel greed, but they do feel greed, and so they work hard to get rid of the feeling. In other words, they try to control the feeling itself as a way of solving the conflict. They think they have to overcome conflict instead of accepting it as normal. Feeling conflict causes tension and anxiety. The impulse is to take control, to try to make it go away.

Ironically, it is only when the conflict is not acknowledged or accepted that it causes more trouble. You tend to act out the feelings or wishes you don't approve of if you don't recognize them. That's because those feelings exist and they will find an outlet some way, somehow. Laying them out on the table where you can see them and name them helps take their power away. Then you can choose whether or not to act on them.

It's similar to the idea that you have to give up trying to control your addiction. "You win by losing," or in other words, you have to be defeated in your efforts to get control before you give up trying. This is as true of trying to control inner conflict as it is of trying to control the addiction itself.

❖

Trying to control conflict does not resolve it. Accepting conflict, accepting responsibility for conflict, and letting go of trying to force resolution may actually resolve it. This is the paradox of "turning it over" that is part of the Twelve Steps.

❖

The Path to the Real Self

At risk of driving you crazy with repetition, developing a real self is the core work of recovery. A woman can only do this by accepting her negative parts, her inner strength, and the internal conflict generated by opposing parts of herself. You get to your real self, your whole, healthy self, by letting yourself feel the heat of your anger as well as the warmth of your kindness. By saying, "I don't want to take care of that other person's needs right now." By saying, "I want," "I need," "I am." If you can allow yourself to hate, you can also love. As you learn to open yourself up to all kinds of feelings, you feel free.

Mai Lee, who used alcohol to escape the anxiety left over from her childhood days when her uncle used to sneak into her bedroom at night, felt at times as if she hated her parents. And she hated the feeling of hating her parents. She was especially angry at her mother. It was her mom's brother who'd been abusive, and she tried once to tell her mom about what was happening. Twenty years later she could still remember the look on her mother's face and the sting in her words. "Mai, your uncle would never do such a thing. You must have been dreaming!" Mai Lee told herself she wasn't angry at her mom; her mom didn't know—couldn't know—and her mom loved her. So this part of the conflict—Mai Lee's hurt and anger at her mother—was largely unconscious for many years.

Yes, her mother did love her, but she had made a devastating error as she wrestled with her own feelings of shock and denial, a mistake that crushed Mai Lee for many years. When Mai Lee finally faced her addiction and entered recovery, she also entered therapy. And here she began to feel safe enough to feel her feelings. She let the anger and resentment she had felt for years bubble to the surface and found herself one day shouting through clenched teeth, "I hate my mother!"

Mai Lee's is a positive story. About four years into recovery, Mai Lee's mother came to therapy with her. She listened to what Mai Lee had to say, and she understood and acknowledged what she'd done. Mai Lee was able to forgive her mother, and they developed a close and loving relationship. Mai Lee had spent many years avoiding the pain of the conflicted feelings, feelings of intense anger and intense need for her mom at the same time. She felt very grateful in therapy for the wholeness she began to feel when she let herself be real. She had no idea that letting herself hate could end up helping her to feel so much love.

Everyone's story does not have such a happy ending of healing in the relationship. But everyone can expand their sense of wholeness when they allow themselves to live with the internal conflict generated by real feelings. Even if the person you are angry at does not accept his or her responsibility for hurting you, you can begin to inhabit your whole and real self when you can accept your own anger. And that can also have a happy ending. Sometimes you can even begin to empathize with and forgive the other person whether or not they get how they hurt you.

Trauma and Internal Conflict

Living with trauma and surviving trauma gives rise to particularly devastating internal conflicts. It leads to the unconscious kind of compromises that Sigmund Freud said we all make, like denying reality. It leads to conscious compromises as well, such as maintaining that the neglect and abuse didn't hurt. As a trauma survivor denies her real feelings along with real events, her real self shuts down and goes into hiding from others and from herself. Being a trauma survivor often means that you carry a lot of secrets about the real you. You carry a secret that you believe you deserved this abuse, and, like Mai Lee, you carry a secret of your anger and your hatred. Your secrets grow bigger; your internal conflicts grow more pressing, and so do your efforts to conceal them.

❀

Accepting and dealing with inner conflict may be particularly important for women early on in recovery if they have lived with trauma. In recovery, they will hear that they are responsible, and it confirms what they've always believed: It was their fault! How do they reconcile this? They were not responsible for being abused as children, but they are responsible for their own drug addictions, which they started as a way of coping with all the pain they felt. How does a woman sort this out? One step at a time.

❀

When Mai Lee had been sober for eight years, she returned to therapy again. She realized she still had a ton of guilt. She felt sick with guilt for every step she made. Her mother developed serious heart disease and was chronically ill. Mai Lee thought she should be supporting her and even living with her. But she didn't want to, and she hated herself for being selfish. She'd ask herself, "Am I responsible for all of this? Am I responsible for her now?" But she felt responsible and had to fight against giving up herself. As we saw, she worked in therapy with her mother when she had four years of sobriety and dealt with her feelings at a deeper level. But now it was very hard to separate out what was being responsible for her own recovery and what she believed she owed her mother. Many women will struggle with this kind of conflict: What, if anything, is "owed," and what is choice?

The Call of Multiple Roles

Living with conflict is terrifically complex. It's hard to recognize and resolve the warring parts of the self or the mixed needs and wishes of yourself and others. In addition to conflict, women also have the complexities of negotiating their multiple roles, such as wife, mother, partner, daughter, sister, professional. There is even ongoing complexity in the recovery path itself. A woman often finds that she is alcoholic and that she is also coalcoholic, or codependent. As she walks her recovery path, she also pays attention to these identities. She begins to go to Al-Anon to address the reality that a husband or partner is an alcoholic. She may identify as an "adult child" too, if her parents were alcoholics. She goes to Adult Children of Alcoholics (ACOA) and Co-Dependents Anonymous (CODA) meetings, finding that this focus helps her open up the trauma issues of her past. How does a woman manage all of this complexity? As we've said before, one step at a time.

A woman in recovery learns to deal with complexity as she learns to be separate and to recognize that there is no such thing as perfection. A woman needs to recognize that her conflict is real, that she does feel divided. And in seeing the reality, she is accountable. She accepts that she feels love and hate at the same time, that she wants to be powerful and to be taken care of at the same time. She begins to recognize that she craves attention, something she always denied, and then she can see that she seeks attention in indirect ways. All kinds of internal and interpersonal conflicts, along with the natural complexities of living, can interfere with treatment and recovery if the woman does not see these conflicts and accept responsibility for them. This is the paradoxical, rugged road to finding her healthy self: Recognizing and accepting the negative with the positive, the conflicts and contradictions, is the only path toward resolution.

Chapter Eight

Independence Built on Dependence

BECOMING SEPARATE THROUGH CONNECTION

Dependence is healthy. "Are you crazy? That's what I'm trying to get rid of," you say. The idea of dependence as healthy can be confusing, especially for people who are addicted and know that *their* dependence is *un*healthy. It's also confusing because so many people hold the idea of dependence in scorn. After all, our belief in our individuality, our self-sufficiency, is the gold standard of American culture. Yet we secretly long to be taken care of. We long to fold ourselves into the caring arms of another so we won't have to feel so self-sufficient. Yes, you may take pride in your power and it feels good, but it doesn't offer the "feeding" that comes with a healthy mutual dependence.

The key here is the phrase *healthy mutual dependence*. The fact is, all people are dependent, and this doesn't have to keep them from being independent. On the contrary, it is what allows them to be independent.

Independence involves a paradoxical acceptance of dependence—a sense that we can't and don't survive alone—along with an understanding that we ultimately stand alone.

✤

Mutual dependence is a curious, baffling mix of seeming opposites. I accept that I am powerless, that I am a limited being, and that I need help. I do not have the power to control my drinking. Yet, at the same time, I must accept responsibility for this lack of power. And the only way I can accept responsibility is to ask for help. I will have to accept my dependence as the route to becoming responsible. That combination is the path to independence.

✤

Independence is not the polar opposite of dependence—you're not a dependent or an independent person, one way or the other—despite the fact that we tend to categorize ourselves along these lines. The woman in recovery comes to see, paradoxically, that being in recovery does not make dependence go away; instead, she makes a shift from unhealthy dependence to healthy dependence. The key change lies in what it is that she is dependent on. She will move from an unhealthy dependence on substances (or her addiction of choice), along with a denial of herself, to an acceptance of her need for dependence, but now, a healthy dependence that will be the foundation for her relationship with herself and others. Her independence is built on her healthy dependence.

The Dependence in Independence

Infant to Adult

In its earliest manifestation, dependence begins in the relationship between an infant and its mother, even before that in-

fant is born. A fetus has a powerful dependence on its mother
to take good care of it so that it can be born with the best possible foundation for healthy development. As we've talked
about earlier, an infant's dependence on its mother is called
an "attachment bond," a connection that is necessary for survival. The attachment grows into a bond of mutual dependence and interdependence as the growing child learns to
communicate its needs to a mother and father who listen,
understand, and respond. Lots of later difficulties in child and
adult development can be traced back to problems in this
early attachment bond with the mother or the father. Physical
and emotional abuse and neglect are typical causes of disrup-
tion that will negatively affect the attachment bond and thus,
the child's development.

Independence grows out of a normal and healthy dependence. How does this happen? In some way, at some time, an
infant's or a child's needs are not met, a reality that will be
true for all of humanity. Parents get it wrong. The attachment
bond is never perfect. Through this bond we hopefully have
experiences of emotional and physical nourishment, of having our needs met directly and correctly, and we'll also have
experiences of frustration. Frustration allows an infant or a
child to develop alternative resources, including herself, to
meet her needs. An infant grows into a girl who can feel
needy and seek help, but who also develops a sense of competence and confidence in herself. It is through the interaction
of dependence and independence that a healthy self can grow.

Dependence + Independence = Interdependence

Though it goes entirely against the grain of what we like to
think, being a healthy, independent adult means having a capacity to be dependent as well. Dependence and independence

together form a healthy interdependence. When a woman is young, she is the most dependent on others to develop her sense of self. As she grows up, she becomes more independent, able to see and to feel herself as separate. When she has a separate, positive sense of herself, she can form close, healthy dependent and interdependent bonds with others, bonds that are not born of unhealthy need.

Unhealthy Dependence

Many, many people get stuck somewhere in this process of healthy development when they form an attachment with a substance or behavior instead of a healthy relationship. People believe that they must meet their needs themselves, instead of reaching out to others in healthy direct ways. So they substitute a substance or behavior, something that helps them think they are meeting their own needs by themselves. Thus begins the road to unhealthy dependence, also called addiction.

❀

Your dependence on your drugs, your overeating or undereating, your smoking, or your gambling served you well in the beginning. It seemed like you had a dependence that worked. It was your greatest security for a long time. It kept you company, and it made bad feelings go away. Never mind that they came back. You just drank some more. You'd probably still be friends with your addiction if it hadn't turned on you.

❀

Addiction is dependence that has gone awry. It's a dependence in which you have sacrificed your self to the power and the dominance of whatever it is you've chosen as your "drug of choice." It might be alcohol, or pot, or food, or it might be your partner. You've given up your separate self in service to this powerful "other." And all the while that you've lost your self and lost your real choice, you believe that this powerful "other" helps you. How? It takes care of you and keeps you from seeing or feeling that you are dependent in any way at all. Yes, that's paradoxical, yet again. You are totally dependent on your drug, a reality that lets you believe that you are not dependent at all!

Distaste for Dependence

Distaste for dependence is central to most addicts. Usually, addicts are independent people. They hate dependence. They're not groupies or dependent whiners. They tend to think of AA as something that's good for people who are weak, for people who can't just stop whenever they want. They pride themselves on self-sufficiency and think if they want to stop drinking, they will just do it themselves without help.

A Bind for Women

All people, for that matter, especially Americans, don't like to be dependent. The American identity is founded on a belief in power, a bootstraps philosophy of self-control. And it is a power that has traditionally resided in the male gender. Women have been assigned the role of dependent, the weaker sex. This gives women's recovery some unique complications. The feminist movement in the late twentieth century, which influenced so many women in one way or another, often left women feeling they had to prove they were equal to men by having power and self-control and by vigorously denying any signs of need.

This was very much the case for Carole. Even in junior high she was concerned with showing others that girls were as capable as boys. And it was exhilarating in college. All around her were opportunities and encouragement, places for a smart, competent woman. A woman could be as powerful as any man. And she did it. She was chief editor of the university's newspaper. And she was scared to death she'd lose it if she showed any signs of weakness. So when she had too many classes, plus her job, and so much pressure she thought she'd crack, she didn't go to anyone for help. She didn't dare say, "I need to cut back on something. Will you help me with this?"

Years later, when she let a serious error pass into publication and had to print a correction, she didn't admit her feeling of vulnerability, her fear that she couldn't really hack it after all. She put her chin in the air and punished the copy editor. When she went back to her apartment that evening, she found herself shaking and grabbed her Vicodin. She couldn't admit to herself or anyone else that she had needs, that she needed help and support from others, that she wasn't totally self-sufficient.

This is a bind. If you acknowledge your dependence, you may believe you're a failure as a feminist, but if you don't acknowledge your dependence, you cannot recover from addiction or become a healthy, mature adult. This is a terrible trap you can get caught in when you struggle to prove yourself "equal" to men in our culture.

Besides, what sounds like the masculine dream actually fits women exactly. If you're not supposed to exist, and if you're not supposed to have needs, wants, or wishes, then how can you feel dependent? It won't work. You must be strong precisely so you can care for everyone else and bear the weight of all that is painful in your family world and in the bigger world too. Recognizing your dependence would be another example of failure.

Control, power, and total self-sufficiency are not healthy goals for either women or men. Acknowledging dependence is a strength, not a weakness, but it's hard for Americans, it's hard for addicts, and it's especially hard for women who are addicted.

What Is Independence?

If we're all dependent, and that's good, then what is independence? What does it mean to be independent if it doesn't mean self-sufficiency? Well, it does mean self-sufficiency to some degree. We are self-sufficient some of the time about some things. But no one is totally self-sufficient. A more accurate word for independence is *autonomy*, a personal freedom that involves an awareness and experience of self as separate from all others. Mature independence is an acceptance of *agency*. That sounds like professional jargon, but it's an important bit of jargon. You are an *agent* in your own life. It says, "I act. I take action. I initiate. I interact." Mature independence also includes an acceptance of responsibility. I am alone and I am responsible, a recognition that can be terrifying.

Unhealthy Independence

Like the concept of dependence, independence can be either unhealthy or healthy. Unhealthy independence is based on a belief in total self-sufficiency. It's a denial of need. It often comes with feelings of grandiosity and omnipotence and an arrogant attitude of superiority. This woman has it made. She's got the answers, and she's got the power.

That's what Carole looked like as she began her climb up the executive ladder, before she tripped on her Vicodin. She was on her way up. She felt full of herself, so sure that she knew everything. She didn't even try to hide her attitude: I'm on the way up and you'd better get out of my path. This led to a false self for Carole, something she had lived with for most of her life. Here's how she described it when she had gotten well into recovery and had the courage and ability to understand where she had been.

> I always had the feeling that "if you knew the real me, you'd run away." I was really a needy gal, a hungry, groveling parasite underneath my facade of independence and control. I pretended that I was strong and didn't need anyone. But deep down, I felt afraid. It was all a charade. I looked good to the world, but I always thought I might crack wide open and end up as a puddle of myself.

Candace is another woman who was convinced that she was independent. She turned tricks, and she was nothing if not independent. On any night of the week as she stood on the street, she could hear a gunshot reverberate somewhere nearby. *So what?* she thought. *That's life. The important thing is that I know how to bring in the money. I know how to take care of myself.*

When she was in jail for the fifth time, she wasn't worried. She knew she'd be out in a couple days, and in the meantime, nobody better touch her. But she was annoyed. One day she was sitting on the couch in the common room with Shenora who wouldn't shut up about treatment.

"When I get outta here, I'm going straight back to the recovery house," Shenora was saying. "Living there with those other women, being straight, it was the best time of my life." Shenora grew up with drugs and gangs and prostitution, so it was a natural progression when she started turning tricks. But she'd gone into treatment and lived in a recovery home for six months before she started using and turning tricks again. "Yeah, girl, you better think about it," Shenora said to Candace.

"I don't need that crap," Candace snapped. "I got control. I only do my drugs when I want to, long after the customers are gone. Maybe you need some cushy recovery home, honey, but not me."

She is one weak woman, Candace thought to herself. *I am never gonna be that needy.* Still, she felt a crack in the shell she'd nurtured since she was a youngster. She'd had a baby when she was seventeen years old. Her mom took care of her son, who was six now, and she missed him while she sat in this damn jail. She started thinking about her son's father. *Wouldn't it be nice . . . Stop it, you idiot,* she scolded herself. *You can't depend on that guy. He might be dead tomorrow. What's the matter with you?*

When Candace entered treatment three years later, it was still very frightening for her to accept how needy she really was.

The kind of "independence" that Carole and Candace had was false. Another name for it is *pseudo-independence.* Pseudo-independence is adopted as a pretense, a defense against feelings of terrible inadequacy, need, and dependence.

The woman who carries this false facade is not self-sufficient at all, though she may convince herself that she is.

In contrast, healthy independence involves an acceptance of both need and responsibility for yourself at the same time. This kind of independence is not based on an inflated belief in self-power. It does not require a facade of false strength. It is an experience of real strength, achieved by accepting your limits.

How Do I Get Healthy Independence?

Remember that healthy independence involves an acceptance of paradox. As individuals alone in the world, we are deeply reliant on others as they are reliant on us. As we accept this responsibility of interdependence, we achieve our paradoxical independence. Autonomy is alone and together.

Geri came to understand this puzzling paradox deeply through the years of her recovery. She was terrified in the beginning when she would be at home in the evening craving her alcohol. Sometimes she would look at John sitting on the couch next to her reading. She wanted to say, "John, take this craving away from me," but he couldn't help. He didn't even get what she felt like. She'd tuck her children into bed and want to snuggle them, thinking somehow that would take away the horrible craving. But the craving was bigger. It grabbed her like a claw and pushed her away from her children.

Then Geri would call her sponsor. In fact, as she jokingly told others, she had five sponsors "to share the load of me." She traded in her alcohol for the women in AA. And it worked. It helped her cope, but it didn't take away the horrible feelings. It was terrifying to know that, no matter whom she called, whom she sat next to, she was bound by this body, this mind. She alone experienced the craving and the terror. No one could lift it off her. She was ultimately alone.

She craved protection like she craved drink. While she couldn't get protection from her feelings, she could get support, and she stuck with it. She called her sponsors often, went to meetings, worked her program. Day by day, minute by minute, she transferred her dependence on her drug to a dependence on her relationship with AA. Eventually, she grew into a deep understanding that she was ultimately alone and she was okay. She was not going to fall apart or fade away. Then one day, finally, she knew. She knew she existed, she was responsible, and she was surrounded by support. She said, "I grew into a feeling of myself alone, and always, together. Now I see that we all do it together. AA is alone, together, and alone-together, with my higher power to hold it all."

Independence is the result of engaging in a healthy developmental process. You can't buy it, you can't get it in a weekend encounter, and you can't even steal it. Independence cannot be bestowed by another, though it can be modeled and fostered. Healthy parents offer their children the secure attachment that will provide the environment and modeling for development that will lead to healthy independence.

This is the same road women take in AA. They make an attachment to recovery—to the people in AA, to the principles of "the program," and ultimately to a higher power. You grow up all over again to become a healthy, autonomous, independent woman, who experiences yourself alone, and together, connected with all others. As in a pomegranate, each woman is a seed, separate in herself, but held in a web of support that makes up a whole community.

Spirituality

How do we talk about spirituality? What is it and why do you find it here in a chapter on dependence and independence? While most people know the word *spirituality* and can talk about what it means to them, it's a distinctly personal word and a distinctly personal experience. You won't find universal agreement about what it is, what it means, or how it works for people, despite the fact that many people talk about spirituality as if it has a universal meaning.

For our purposes here, I'll define spirituality in a very distinct way, as it fits within a developmental view. Spirituality means dependence. Spirituality is the acceptance of one's basic, fundamental need for an "other." It's a need we've defined as attachment so far, the bond between an infant and a mother and father, or caregiver, which "holds" and gratifies the child's needs and provides the structure for on-going healthy development. This bond of healthy dependence is the vehicle for the child to develop into a healthy, separate grown-up.

We've looked at how healthy development goes astray when you shift your deepest emotional investment from a healthy relationship with an "other" to a substitute. You become invested in the substance, behavior, or unhealthy relationship that feels like it meets your needs and solves your emotional conflicts. This is your new attachment, your new dependence, in fact, your addiction. In a sense, your addiction becomes your higher power. Your spirituality is your unhealthy dependence. It is the one thing that is greater than yourself that you think you can trust. Yet, instead of protecting you, it destroys you. Your false "higher power" of alcohol, other drugs, food, or your lover can't do the job. Eventually it doesn't work. This distortion of a higher power turns on you. Hitting bottom is the deep, face-to-face encounter with the failure of your attachment, your unhealthy dependence.

In recovery, your spirituality is your new healthy dependence, your relationship with other people, with yourself, with a higher power. You may name your higher power whatever term makes sense to you, but at bottom it's a relationship with a nurturing, supportive "other," an other that is greater than the self or any person. This is something we will take a closer look at in the next chapter.

Trauma and Independence

Women who have experienced trauma have a difficult time traveling the road to independence. This includes all women in recovery, because the experience of being out of control is itself a trauma. Addiction is trauma. In addition, many, perhaps most, women in recovery have also been victimized at the hands of another.

This trauma makes traveling the road to independence difficult for all women in recovery. They may well maintain abstinence, but they struggle with the Steps and their acceptance of inherent dependence. These women want to arrive at autonomy without relying on anyone or anything. They may get Step One only too well. "Yes, I am powerless." But they balk at Step Two. They cannot "come to believe" in a higher power that will restore them to sanity. Here begins resistance to recovery for so many women.

Why? Because dependence has hurt these women badly. Lack of power is all many women have known. Unfortunately, the overly dependent role women have been assigned in our society makes them vulnerable to being victimized. They were kids, trusting an abusive parent. They were adult women, trusting an abusive partner. They were teens, catapulted into adult womanhood and adult sexuality. They were traumatized in trusting relationships, so they experience intense inner conflict about granting authority to anything higher than their own self-power.

❀

A woman who has experienced trauma often develops a kind of self-sufficiency that is not based on grandiosity, but on a need for protection. Her self-sufficiency isn't based on a sense that she is powerful and strong, but on the opposite, on the deep sense that she cannot rely on others for anything, and that it is dangerous to do so. So she works to overcome this state of helplessness.

❀

Remember, resisting a sense of helplessness is a natural instinct for all women in recovery, and doubly so for women who have been traumatized by others. These women survive by withdrawing into themselves. If they are dependent only on themselves, they don't have to face the knowledge that they need others, a knowledge that is terrifying in the face of how they feel hurt by others. And then, when they lost control to their addiction, they discovered that they couldn't even trust themselves. What's more, they have to face how they have caused their own trauma. Whether or not a woman has been victimized by a trusted other or has been traumatized by her own addiction, her own actions, she has to face this reality.

Women who have been traumatized by others often report that they survived a terrible experience by withdrawing into themselves and by "going out of their bodies." They describe removing themselves perceptually and emotionally from the horrific "now" by dissociation, placing themselves outside of the real experience. It is a mechanism of survival. When a woman feels trapped by the reality of a threatening "other," or by the memory of threat that she now carries within her, she shuts off and she shuts down. She "goes away."

Unfortunately, she also ends up "going away" from people who can help her. This kind of withdrawal is such a total dependence on the self that it prohibits the possibility of emotional connection with others. This kind of self-sufficiency is called an "autistic self" by professionals. It's not the same thing as autism, a disorder of withdrawal. Yet it means something similar. It is such a severe withdrawal that it becomes a lived experience of being alone. When a real dependency relationship has been destructive, or has been thwarted, the woman creates her own "other," which is herself. This "other" may be her inner voice; it may feel like it's a part of her, or it may feel like it's outside, a kind of omniscient presence that warns her of danger. But the bottom line is that she reaches "in," not "out," for help.

While this adaptation helped her survive living with dangerous others she couldn't control, and becoming a danger to herself through her own addiction, it also keeps her from experiencing a healthy dependence that will lead her to a healthy self. She may struggle with dependence all through her process of recovery growth. She inches her way toward accepting her dependence and allowing herself to open to the outside, to the presence and help of others.

These women often survive the hurdles and conflicts of recovery by relying on the old "false self," side by side with the growth of the new, healthy self. They may consciously feel an "old me" and a "new me." They can accommodate both selves quite well, letting the "new me" hold strong in recovery while the "old me" intrudes all along the way. This is the normal course. The "old you" is also the "child within," the young woman or girl who lived in fear of others and comes alive in recovery to warn the grown-up woman that she should be careful, that trusting others will lead to danger, harm, and death.

Often, the structure of AA and the guidelines of the Steps provide reassurance. A woman is not "turning over" her self to control by any "other." She must do the work herself. Still, she trusts in the experience of others, and she trusts in the bigger and greater power of AA. It's a new kind of dependence. It's not the loss of her self at all. It's a claim of self and a trust that others will show her how to grow and how to survive. She does not depend on anyone to take over for her. She does not give up her autonomy and her newfound responsibility. She starts recovery by a claim of self, by saying yes to powerlessness, yes to abstinence, and yes to her need for help. Then she takes the steps that will lead to maturity and healthy independence. This is responsibility.

In this process, she may come to feel saved by the idea of a higher power. She can come to a deep experience of trust, perhaps not yet in people, but in a power greater than herself and greater than any human. This has been the route to responsibility and freedom for many women.

As we've seen before, Mai Lee really struggled with this issue. She felt the danger of depending on others acutely when she entered AA. At first she was unable to even allow herself to ask for a sponsor. There was an older woman in the group whom she found comforting. Her eyes showed gentle, inviting laugh lines whenever she smiled. Mai Lee had almost decided she would ask her, but as she talked with her, she heard a voice in her head criticizing the woman. *Maybe she isn't that nice,* Mai Lee thought. Then there was another woman, just barely older than Mai Lee herself, who came to each meeting looking great. Mai Lee thought how much she'd like to be like her. *I'll bet she can relate to me,* Mai Lee thought. But each time she tried to ask her to be her sponsor, her stomach would tighten. The voice in her head said, *Mai, she thinks she's classier than you.* Although Mai Lee didn't understand it at the time, relying on a sponsor felt too intimate and too dangerous.

After about five months of meetings, Mai Lee was struck by the word *God* when another woman was talking about relying on her higher power. She had believed in God growing up. She figured there just had to be a reason for all this, even if she couldn't know what it was. But she knew somehow that it was God who got her to AA. That's what really saved her in the beginning. She could trust in God, and she didn't have to depend on anyone. As she watched God work through the people in AA, she learned by watching them. Eventually she became better at trusting people, but, as she explained to a frightened newcomer at a meeting years later, "It's a new meaning of trust. You take care of you, and I take care of me, and we support each other."

Mai Lee was describing interdependence. We stand alone, and we stand together. This combination of individual autonomy and responsibility, coupled with shared learning and support, defines our final paradox: learning to learn from others in order to stand alone, together.

In summary, women who are addicted have an unhealthy dependence, a dependence that is total and leaves them without a self. In recovery, this is switched to a healthy dependence—the kind of dependence that is unavoidably part of being human, the need for others. This doesn't mean you don't have a separate self, only that you can't live a whole life alone. It's like the dabs of paint in an impressionist painting. Each one is separate in and of itself. But it can't make the painting alone. It needs all the other dots to make a whole painting.

You enter the path to recovery by acknowledging your unhealthy dependence *and* your legitimate need for dependence. You enter the path to independence by practicing healthy dependence. When you can know and accept the need you have for others, you can also fill the need in healthy, direct ways that allow you to take responsibility for yourself and allow you to develop a separate, autonomous self. This is healthy independence. Interdependence.

So begins the journey of transformation. Women in recovery come to grasp the new truth: You have to accept and experience dependence to know independence.

Chapter Nine

Standing Alone with the Help of Others

THE APPRENTICE MODEL OF AA
AND OTHER TWELVE STEP GROUPS

You know by now that recovery is all about growing your new self, and you know that the process is filled with paradoxes. In accepting that you are powerless, you gain the ability to become a responsible, strong woman. In accepting the reality of conflict, of internal division, you become a mature, whole woman. In accepting the depths of your human dependence, you are able to gain a healthy independence. You know what it means to be alone and to feel connected with others at the same time.

Connection is critical through all of this; you come to know yourself deeply by being open to learn from others. In other words, you find your separate self through your relationship with others. This isn't a "turning over" of yourself to the care and protection of other people. It isn't giving up yourself to someone else's authority. No, it's something quite different. It is a reliance on others for support and encouragement, for guidance, for showing the way, while you remain responsible for yourself. You rely on others, but you are responsible for taking care of yourself. This is the paradox we will talk about here. It is also the foundation of AA and other Twelve Step groups. You learn to learn from others so you can stand alone, on your own two feet.

Wanting Someone to Take Over

Like the idea of healthy dependency, the idea of relying on others at the same time that you're responsible for yourself may seem confusing. There's a distinction here between relying on others and having them take care of you. You may feel like you want to return to that infant state where somebody else just does it all for you. But that's not what you need. Not really. You need others to hang in there with you while they show you how to take care of yourself. Ironically, you need others to take care of themselves so you can learn how to take care of yourself.

This is what is called the *apprentice model* of AA.[1] This model validates a woman's fundamental autonomy and her inherent dependence on others. You need the other women in AA to work their own programs. You need them to focus on themselves and not take over for you, even though taking over might be exactly what you think you want.

You remember Sharifa. We first met Sharifa in chapter 2, Sharifa who ignored all her own needs in favor of taking care of everybody else, and who then turned to midnight ice-cream binges. She also turned to midafternoon brownie binges and

1. This brief interpretation of AA is the author's point of view. For a more detailed perspective, readers are encouraged to explore AA literature, such as the book *Twelve Steps and Twelve Traditions* (New York: Alcoholics Anonymous World Services, 1996).

midmorning sweet rolls. She slowly and despairingly grew out of each new size of clothing, and her husband, Barack, began nagging her about her weight. Her doctor nagged her too. Sharifa began her recovery in Overeaters Anonymous (OA).

It was hard to go, but she felt enormous relief when she walked through the door and sat down at her first meeting. Somehow she thought it would be like a magic pill; she could relax and let somebody else take over for her. She left the meeting about 9:30 P.M. thinking, *That wasn't so hard.* When she got home Barack wanted her to iron his shirt for the next day. Tired as she was by this time, she set up the ironing board and was interrupted by a call from her sister who wanted to talk about problems with her son's teacher. She spent thirty minutes brainstorming ideas with her sister then ironed Barack's shirt. By 10:30 P.M. she was exhausted, feeling an irritation she didn't want to feel, and wouldn't you know it? An ice cream binge. The same night she went to her first OA meeting. Although Sharifa wouldn't have put it this way, it was her first lesson that no one else could stop eating for her. Over the years she came to rely on others to show her how they did it and to support her as she stopped overeating. But she had to be responsible for herself.

What Is the Apprentice Model of AA?

In the apprentice model of AA and other Twelve Step programs, you learn to learn from others. This happens in a variety of ways and at various speeds as well. There are many ways to be involved in AA, but basically, the apprentice model involves, first of all, attachment, and then learning and teaching.

Attachment

We've talked a lot about attachment throughout this book. Attachment comes at the very beginning of life; it is at the core of being human. A healthy attachment in our early years carries us throughout our lives and makes it possible for us to trust others enough to get—and give—the help and support all people need.

Attachment is also at the beginning of AA. As you know so well, women who are addicted have formed an overriding attachment to a substance, behavior, or person. It is the unhealthy dependence we explored in the last chapter. In AA women transfer their unhealthy attachment to the healthy attachment of Twelve Step meetings, symbols, wisdom, and direction, and to the other women in recovery. In the beginning, attachment to AA is all about dependence, and that's okay.

Early on in AA a woman often feels great need, just like the infant we learned about in the early chapters of this book. She needs a protective parent, a parent who provides safety for her in which to take shelter. AA literally and figuratively "holds" her intense dependency needs as she begins to feel calm and safe sitting in a meeting or talking on the phone.

Don't be afraid to ask for all the help you need in Twelve Step groups. Your dependence here is not unhealthy. You will learn that you can't feed yourself too much of AA. You should go to meetings all the time, reach out to quiet a craving, calm a frustration, or fill an internal hole. As a woman reaches out, she is "cradled" and rocked through the early days of anxiety and need. She can then build her healthy self on the foundation of this healthy dependence.

✤

This is one of the paradoxes of AA: The meetings, the people, and the program are designed to accept human dependence and to gratify human need, a process that becomes the foundation for healthy development of self and of self-with-other. Over time, you will learn how to find your own self and trust yourself such that dependence and independence find a balance.

✤

Learning

Another basic element in the AA model is learning. The woman in recovery depends on others who have come before her in active addiction and recovery to show her and teach her how to recover. You can't learn this alone. Yes, you have to look inward to find yourself, but not in isolation. It is through the help of another who shows you the way that you can proceed with the development of your new self. If you try to do this alone, if you look for the "answers" only from within yourself, you will find the merry-go-round you already know. You will find your false self, ready to greet you with all your defenses.

Teaching

Teaching is just as important as learning in AA. In fact, you can't really take the learning and the teaching apart. In the Twelve Step program, a woman is always a learner and always a teacher. The relationships are reciprocal. Even the women who have been in recovery for many, many years will find themselves learning from the women who have just entered recovery. This is the way of recovery, of Twelve Step participation. Everyone is on this journey; every woman is a learner; every woman is dependent on others, just like you are. Every woman is also a teacher. No matter how long a woman has been in recovery, she has her own experience to share, an experience that will be recognizable—known deeply—to another.

The combining of learner and teacher is a developmental process. In the initial attachment phase, when a woman is busy absorbing so much new learning, she likely feels needy and scared, clearly the one who is the "helpee." She doesn't feel like a teacher at all. But even at this stage, she is helping others. She is helping them by the very fact of her newness. By showing up and asking for help, she reminds others where they have come from. It's a constant remembering, a sharing that confirms for everyone the realities of the past and their commitment to recovery and the present.

When Sharifa first went to her meetings, she felt like the new kid on the block. For Sharifa, this was also a blessing because it gave her permission not to take care of anybody else. How could she be expected take to care of others when she was the new one and didn't know what she was doing yet? But she was surprised to find that other people came up to her, even at the first meeting, and thanked her for coming. They told her it helped them to hear her learning to stay abstinent. *Yeah, right,* she thought. *They're just being polite.*

She didn't believe them at first, but after she'd been in the program awhile, she started to understand what they meant. As she was listening to Bonnie, a newcomer, talk, Sharifa felt a surge of gratitude to the trembling, young woman whose courage was evident in her effort to introduce herself. She felt inspired again a couple of meetings later by some wise words Bonnie offered. *This must be what they were talking about when I first came,* she thought. *Nobody's ever got it all wrapped up.*

How Does It All Work Together?

How do attachment, learning, and teaching take place? It takes place in the meetings, in the comfort and guidance of the words repeated at each meeting, and in the support of peers. It takes place in the mentoring relationship of a sponsor. It takes place in relationships. It takes place ultimately and most profoundly in your relationship with a higher power.

From Isolation to Connection

At first you depend on your peers and elders in AA. The people in AA can be substitute "parents." They teach the "child of recovery" new behavior and new language that help you shift your dependence away from yourself and your drug onto others, the program of AA, and to a new higher power.

A woman might come to a meeting, however quietly or tentatively, and sit in a room with other women who have walked this path before her, as well as with other women just taking their first steps. As she participates in the ritual words of the opening, as she listens to other people speak of their experience, and as she gathers the courage to connect by offering her own words, she begins to form relationships. But how far and how fast, how close and how quickly, varies greatly from woman to woman.

Each Woman Has Her Own Timing

Some women quickly form close bonds with other recovering women. This intense bond of shared experience provides an immediate attachment of security for the woman who is newly dry and recognizes that she doesn't know how to stay abstinent and become sober.

Some women can't form any kind of relationship yet. They may experience a need for distance: They intentionally maintain a space between themselves and others. In that space, they can tentatively approach and retreat from abstinence and recovery with a sense of guarding their own safety. They can make an attachment to recovery, but not yet to any people in recovery.

As we've talked about in the last chapter, many women who have experienced trauma are intensely wary and frightened of relationships of any kind and especially a relationship that seems to promise help. These women felt repeatedly betrayed by the promise of closeness and help earlier in their lives, and they're not about to jump in without a lot of testing. Many people also have learned from their parents that they were bad in some way. If their parents were troubled, unhealthy, perhaps addicted themselves, they were able to give their children only negative feeling and awful words. And so they are wary as they begin to form new attachments in AA.

Candace went for a whole year to NA meetings before she really began to form an attachment to the other women there. She was used to taking care of herself and her son, and she wanted to do this recovery thing for herself too. Yeah, she knew she was powerless, but she had no idea how people could help her. To her, help always meant shame.

Her mother's help had always come with a lecture. Her mother took care of Candace's son every day, but she never failed to tell Candace each morning that she was stupid, that she'd never amount to anything. So Candace knew her inability to quit using crack was all because she was stupid. She hated that she didn't know how to leave it alone.

She kept going back and forth at meetings between wanting to listen and being furious. It didn't matter what the other women said to her. She kept hearing her mother's criticism and loathing coming from everybody in the room. Her inner voice said, *Girl, you're a goner.* Her stomach tightened at the thought of letting anyone in close.

So Candace hung back and watched. Slowly, as she saw how these women took care of themselves and took responsibility for their own behavior, even the using, she began to understand how she could do that too. But she could never have stayed in the program if she had to tell a lot about herself or get really close to people early on.

Sharifa wasn't really like that. She jumped in from the first meeting. Even though she felt skeptical when the others told her she was helping them too, it felt good to her, and she was quick to put her whole self into the meeting. She felt attached to the other women from practically the first meeting on. Women's pacing differs enormously. You can make your attachments at whatever pace feels right to you.

However slowly, however quickly, you *will* begin to form attachments in AA. And the relationships are formed through sharing experiences. In fact, this is the standard operating procedure in Twelve Step meetings. *One individual teaches another by sharing her experience.* She shows the newcomer how to do it by modeling recovery actions and sharing her "story," what people in Twelve Step programs call her "experience, strength, and hope." In AA language, the woman both "talks the talk" and "walks the walk."

"Talking the Talk"

Telling your story is central to AA, telling your story as it used to be and telling your story as it grows, day by day. The woman in AA tells "what it was like, what happened, and what it is like now" that she is in recovery.

"What it was like" is the story of active addiction. She tells what it was like for her, what she thought and what she did while she was drinking, using, eating, gambling, or locked into an obsessive, unhealthy relationship. It's a story about the loss of control—what I did, how it felt, and what I was thinking that kept it going.

"What happened" is the story of the end of the line. It's the tale of the downward spiral into the pit of utter despair and helplessness. For the woman in recovery, it's eventually the point of surrender, the moment when she faces herself and knows that she has lost control and that she is responsible— alone—for "what happened."

"What it is like now" is the story of recovery. The woman who has ten minutes has a story of ten minutes of abstinence. The woman then has one day, two days, a week, a month, and then she comes to one year. On she goes if she is in solid recovery. She will have a deepening story of her active addiction, and she will have a longer, deepening story of her recovery. She tells the story of her false, addicted self and of her journey to become her real self in recovery. This is the ongoing story, the one that becomes new every day.

"Walking the Walk"

Veterans in recovery also show the newly recovering woman "how it works" by modeling their program of recovery. This is where "what you do" matters so much. A woman in AA provides a model of recovery for others. A woman new in recovery recognizes herself through listening to the stories of others. She depends on them to show her the way. She depends on other women in recovery to "show up," to stay sober, and to develop into healthy recovering women *themselves*. The woman in recovery—the newly sober woman and the woman who came before her—grows more and more into her own ability to be real and to acknowledge herself by hearing and seeing others do exactly that.

The Parts of a Twelve Step Program

The Meetings

Most commonly, people begin their participation in AA or other twelve step groups by attending meetings. Here is where you start to build the relationships that will sustain you. Meetings are opened by the ritual of reading the Steps. This reading of the Steps provides both encouragement and guidance, and it eventually becomes a comfort the instant you hear it as you begin to associate it with the comfort of the meeting. It is at meetings that you meet other women and men going through the same thing you are going through and where you share your stories. But you can speak or not speak at a meeting as you will. Meetings also provide an opportunity to provide what's called "service," making coffee, serving as a secretary for the meetings, or serving as a sponsor.

Sometimes conditions don't permit human contact. Women may live in a rural area or suffer from disabilities that make attendance at meetings difficult. These women can establish a relationship through books and pamphlets, and now through the computer. They can attend meetings online. The key is the move from isolation to engagement, from a reliance on self alone to a self with other.

The Sponsor

The sponsor is another important part of AA. The sponsor is like a personal tutor who introduces you to recovery—to the new behaviors, the language, and the work of the Steps. The sponsor is a mentor, the one who shows you the ropes.

Geri had a sponsor before she completed the intensive part of treatment. Her sponsor was a bridge for her from the sheltered world of spending the day in treatment to the bigger world of recovery. Having a sponsor made a huge difference at her first meeting. When Geri's sponsor met her at the door and welcomed her to the meeting, an image flashed in her mind of the time when she and John had just moved to their neighborhood. A lovely woman had rung their doorbell and welcomed them with pamphlets and coupons and a list of services and phone numbers that Geri and John might need early on. When Geri was much further along in recovery, she could appreciate this image in a way she wasn't able to at the time. *I didn't find coupons in AA, but my temporary sponsor welcomed me to the neighborhood,* she thought as she chuckled to herself. It was easier to stay on the AA block with that kind of support. Geri found a regular sponsor fairly soon, but she has kept in touch with her first mentor through all her years in recovery.

Many women start immediately with a temporary sponsor, like the welcome woman or a buddy at camp. After a while, she may ask this temporary person to be her permanent sponsor, or she may seek a different woman to guide her in her ongoing recovery work. Some women have only one sponsor for their recovery lifetimes, and others have many. Each woman finds her own best way to be an apprentice, to be a learner with a mentor in recovery. And then she becomes a teacher too, a mentor for another woman on this recovery road. And so it goes, woman to woman.

Ups and Downs in Relationships with Sponsors

Are these attachments to recovery mentors perfect? Well, of course not.

Because other people in AA are human too, they cannot be a woman's new higher power. It's not even guaranteed that they'll be healthy parents. A woman's peers and the woman she chooses for a sponsor will be fallible too. They're bound to be as they're on the same journey she is. So a woman will likely learn from many women and men as she grows in recovery. She will take what she needs from whomever has what she needs at the moment. She will find stable, healthy women and men who show her "how it works" for them, and she will encounter unhealthy women and men who are not a help to her. Luckily, there are a lot of substitute "parents" and peers to choose from.

A sponsor's human imperfections, as well as the imperfections of other peers, actually offer you opportunities. They let you reexperience the patterns of your earliest bonds with family that were difficult and learn new ways of relating. Your earliest experiences as a baby, toddler, and growing child will reappear, sometimes wildly and obviously and sometimes with subtle hints.

You remember Mai Lee and the difficulty she had trusting

others. After she had been in AA for a year or so, she began to pull away from her sponsor and friends. She'd go to a meeting, and during the coffee time before the meeting started, she'd see Jennifer and Lea laughing together. She'd see Latoya and Gloria checking their meeting schedules and making a coffee date. Everybody seemed to be so close to each other, and it seemed like nobody ever sought her out. One day she was standing on the edge of the room when she spotted her sponsor on the other side. With a rush of relief, she walked over to her, knowing at least her sponsor would make a point of talking to her. But her sponsor just nodded a quick hello and continued with the conversation she'd been having. After that, Mai Lee began to call her sponsor less and less.

Finally, her sponsor called her and asked what was going on. As they talked, Mai Lee began to realize that she was feeling at the meetings the same way she used to feel in her school when she was a child, like the odd person out. It dawned on her that she was repeating childhood patterns. She didn't want to isolate herself in recovery as she had when she was a child, so she decided to take a closer look inside. That's when she began work on the Fourth Step, which she had been resisting.

As a woman stabilizes in her recovery and begins to work the Steps, she can reflect on her attachment to the program, on what she hears, sees, and knows, and let these new insights move her to internal exploration. And as time goes on and she feels secure in her attachment to her sponsor, to her friends, to the structure of the program, she'll find she can tolerate looking inside. A woman can find herself replaying unhealthy, old patterns at any point in recovery. They will undoubtedly crop up more than once, more than twice, more than several times, each time presenting an opportunity to learn and grow. The security a woman feels in her attachments to her sponsor, her friends, and the structure of the program, as well as a woman's own work on the Steps, will guide her and allow her real self to emerge.

Higher Power

The woman can look at herself deeply because her ongoing process of growth is ultimately structured and contained by a deepening relationship with her higher power. It is this "higher other" that protects all women in recovery. The higher power that each woman constructs for herself ensures that all women in the Twelve Step program will be equal. They will always be both learners and teachers. No one outgrows being a learner.

You will remember from our discussion of spirituality in the last chapter that spirituality can be described as a healthy dependence, a dependence that soothes and feeds and provides the structure and environment for new development. A woman transfers her unhealthy addictive dependence to a healthy higher power that she rediscovers, or that she creates, through the process of her development. But not everybody finds this easy.

Candace thought the idea of a higher power was "crap." Even after two years of meetings, she had said to a friend, "This 'God thing' is going to drive me crazy." Her mother had preached God at her all the time, preached God in the same breath that she told Candace she'd never amount to anything. "You gotta get God in your life, honey, or you won't amount to a hill of beans," she'd nag her. As far as Candace was concerned, God didn't amount to a hill of beans. God didn't seem to give two hoots that her life was a mess.

Still, she knew she needed NA, so she just sort of let the

"God stuff" be. As she continued to go and to see how she could trust the others to hang in there with her, she began to trust that there was someone or something out there that cared about her in this world. She began to trust that there was someone or something that spoke to her in that still, small voice inside. There were others in her meeting who called their higher power God, and others who talked about the universal energy. What Candace came to understand is that she was in charge of what she believed in. There is not one God out there—the AA God—that you have to buy. It's personal, and you have to find your own. But the bottom line is it can't be you!

A higher power provides equality for the woman to flourish in an apprentice relationship. It is the structure of this relationship that provides the opportunity for healthy dependence that will grow into healthy independence, autonomy, and interdependence, an experience of self based on responsibility and connection.

In summary, the way the apprentice model of AA and other Twelve Step programs works is by giving women who are addicted a healthy substitute for their unhealthy substance or behavior. In AA, the woman who is addicted can find a new healthy "object" for her attachment, and in this new relationship, she can find the support and wisdom and guidance to grow into her self.

In AA she listens to the stories of others and watches as they go about the business of taking care of themselves. As she learns from watching and listening, she develops her own story and builds her healthy self in a continuing, open-ended way. This she in turn shares with others, and in the sharing, she teaches. She also teaches by her presence from the very beginning. She is an equal partner, giving and receiving, from the moment she walks in the door, whether she knows it or not. In the nurture and challenge of her peers, her sponsor, her higher power, and the guidance of the program, the woman can dare to discover her real self.

But she is not headed for a "graduation" of any kind, nor is she looking to the day when she can finish this hard work. Her outlook now is different. She is living the result of her transformation. She's not focused on getting control. She's not still longing for the power she always wanted. She is involved in a developmental process that does not end. She never stops growing and learning. She does grow up, and she does grow healthy, but this growth is not leading her to a destination of self-sufficiency. She now lives in connection. She is always learning and she is always teaching as she shares her self with others in recovery.

PART FOUR

At Home in Recovery

Chapter Ten

The Gifts of Recovery

A woman in recovery gets what she wanted. She gains the fundamental rights, entitlements, attitudes, values, freedoms, and responsibilities that she always longed for, envied, or feared, but usually not in the way, shape, or form that she always imagined. Her gifts of maturity only come to her as a result of being in recovery and of doing the developmental work. The gifts of recovery don't arrive fully formed on her doorstep the moment she decides she wants to try to get sober. They grow slowly along with her, until one day, after many years of immersing herself in learning and practicing the developmental steps of recovery, she realizes she is living a full and rich life. She has received gifts she couldn't even dream of before. What are those gifts?

Goals and Aspirations

The woman in recovery has goals and aspirations of her own. Recovery gives you the right to a separate self and the responsibility to grow that self. And this in turn lets you think about who you are, what you want, and how to get it. You know you can plan—must plan—even though you can't control the results. You know how to balance thinking about yourself with thinking about others. You know how to give and take, to compromise. Most of the time, you can "wear the world as a loose garment" and it feels like the right size. You get a new kind of control you never dreamed possible. This is what allows you to have realistic aspirations and to know the steps you must take to achieve your goals.

When women have been in recovery long enough to feel some security, they often begin to recognize that they have wishes, skills, and talents and allow themselves to step out into the world with them. They have the security to pursue interests that don't focus on recovery, but are born of recovery, and the ability to set goals and plans to make them happen. This is what happened to Geri.

Geri had dreamed of being a writer since long before she entered recovery, but she thought it was totally beyond her reach. Often, when the kids were very young and taking their naps, she'd sit at the kitchen counter and write, maybe the beginning of a story, maybe a poem. But she'd stop after about fifteen minutes. *This stuff is awful,* she'd tell herself. *I can't write worth a dime.* And she'd head for a drink. She'd read about a class at the community center on how to write magazine articles and thought how much she'd like to do that. But she was scared to death of taking one, sure she'd make a fool of herself.

When Geri had been in recovery for seven years, she found she had more confidence in herself, and she decided to take one of those classes at the community center. The class confirmed her desire to be a writer and boosted her belief that she could do it. By this time in recovery, Geri had gained the ability to form goals, and she decided she wanted to try her hand at journalism. She had also gained the ability to plan. She talked with John, and they decided together that they could afford for her to take classes part time at the university when the children were in school. She figured that by the time they were teenagers, she would have her bachelor of arts degree and could look for a job in journalism.

When Geri had been in recovery twelve years, she had indeed earned her degree and gotten her first job as a journalist. Geri had experienced recovery's gift of having goals and aspirations. She also experienced many other gifts that went into her new career path.

A Sense of Mastery

Mastery is a sense of internal competence. It's a sense of security, a sense of trust that you're on the right track. Mastery is one of the roots of positive self-esteem. It is a competency born and grown from within. I've talked all the way through this book about developmental stages, about how you first need a healthy dependence and from this you can develop a separate sense of self that can act. This is what mastery is based on. It's the normal developmental path of childhood and the normal developmental path of recovery.

People sometimes confuse the idea of mastery with control, but mastery has nothing to do with "getting control." On the contrary, mastery is about knowing what you can do and having confidence in that. Part of mastery for Geri was daring to take a writing course and discovering that she could, in fact, do it and do it well. As she recognized her ability to study and write and learn, she gained the confidence to pursue her dream.

Mastery is what you get when you stop fighting for control, seek help, and stay open to learn through others. When you have mastery, you know you can tackle and solve problems, and you know there are things you cannot do. Mastery is something like "the wisdom to know the difference" from the Serenity Prayer. Mastery offers the great pleasure of feeling yourself to be competent, skilled, bright, funny, charming, and sure at the same time that you can be brittle, caustic, angry, and naughty. This is all of you.

Strength and Stamina

The woman in recovery has an abiding experience of inner strength. She has survived trauma, and she is intact and feels more deeply grounded than she ever has in her life. This isn't because she knows she can control things or because she is sure everything will come out the way she wants it. Rather, it's because she knows, with the help of others and her higher power, she can cope. Her stamina comes from giving over the source of power to a higher authority. Her strength is not a "power over" anybody, though she could easily derail herself by thinking of it this way. Rather, it is the true experience of empowerment, and she can *only* know it by growing into it through her own hard work. And once again, this deep strength and stamina are the results of her developmental work.

Part of the gift you get from this kind of strength is knowing you can't be all or do all. Nobody is that powerful. Knowing your limits is the great source of self-acceptance, and it gives you great freedom and responsibility. Freedom offers limitless possibility, with a responsibility to make choices, often called the "burden of choice." It is the action of choice that confirms the limits.

When Geri had been at the university for two years, her

best friend was diagnosed with a life-threatening illness. Geri couldn't control the outcome. She could only spend time with her, support her, love her. Not only did she spend a lot of time with her friend, but she thought about her a lot. She was distracted, and it hurt her studies. But Geri continued to work her program and rely on her higher power. And at that point, after her nine years in sobriety, she never seriously doubted that she had the inner strength to cope with whatever happened. Fortunately, Geri's friend recovered, and Geri got her classes back on track. But she knew she would have found the strength and stamina to live with whatever happened.

Accepting Emotion

The woman in recovery has the pleasure of feeling and expressing her emotions instead of trying to control them, hide them, or get rid of them. In fact, knowing, feeling, and expressing your emotions allows you to maintain your sobriety and to live in a solid, positive relationship with yourself and others. You no longer have to hide from yourself or others the anger, rage, or selfishness you sometimes feel. You might not express everything you feel, but you know it doesn't prove you're a bad person. Accepting your emotions lets you live with clarity. Instead of being overwhelmed by confusion, you let yourself recognize what you feel and then figure out what it's about with a trusted other, such as your sponsor or therapist. You get to choose what, when, and whether you share.

In the early days of recovery, you probably felt overwhelmed by your emotions. The first time Geri really let herself cry, she cried so much she felt like she had a hangover the next day. But over time, you come to know you will survive all kinds of feelings, from joy to devastation, from love to rage. And it feels wonderful. It feels wonderful to be able to cry deeply, or let your anger out, or laugh with abandon.

It gives you a bigger sense of yourself, and you grow bigger inside. It lets you connect with yourself, and it lets your real self connect with others.

Belonging

The woman in recovery finds her real self, and this lets her connect with others. She gets the joy of having a sense of belonging. In early recovery, you probably struggled with the polar opposites of needing to belong in order to "fix" yourself but being afraid that you'd lose yourself if you belonged. As you mature in recovery, you see that belonging has nothing to do with giving up yourself. It's the opposite. You can only belong when you relate to others from your real self.

The themes of "fitting in" and "belonging" are important for all women because relationship is so central to a woman's experience of herself. As we've seen throughout this book, it's often harder for a woman to think about herself alone, herself as separate, than it is to think about herself with others. Women so often have had to give up their "selves" in order to belong. In recovery, you first find a self and then you can belong, but now it's a belonging that feels true and right.

Respect for Self

The woman in recovery has developed respect for her self and for her needs, wants, and wishes, and she receives respect from others in return. When you come to know yourself deeply and accept yourself, you don't have to live your life looking for approval from others. You don't need permission from others to feel what you feel or behave as you choose to behave. Again, this is freedom. It is exhausting always to look over your shoulder, to monitor the reactions of others and then decide who you should be. In recovery, you gain the self-respect that allows you to feel and be your separate self. You live with a deep respect for yourself that guides you in all your actions.

This deep self-respect lets you work through your relationships with others. You may face difficult times with your partner, your family, and your friends and colleagues as you grow yourself in recovery. If others do not change, you may face a rougher road of recovery and very hard choices down the line. But above all, you get to like yourself, live comfortably with yourself, and then you can build relationships that are rewarding. No one can give you the gift of self-respect. You grow into it.

A Healthy Self

A healthy self. This is what you can expect in recovery, and this is the big gift of recovery. This is all of the other gifts put together. A healthy self is what you have worked so hard to claim and to build. You will know that all the paradoxes of recovery have given you a self and allowed you to grow into a strong, secure, and trusting relationship with yourself, your higher power, and all the "others" in your life. You will laugh as you happily tell a friend that you are powerless in every aspect of your life, and as a result, you've never been better, never felt stronger, and never trusted so deeply. You will chuckle when you note that you didn't achieve this happy state all by yourself, that you're a very dependent person, and you don't ever want to be self-sufficient again. Not that you ever really were, mind you. You just thought you should be.

But don't worry, you'll reassure others; even though you're dependent, you're responsible for meeting your needs. It will all make sense to you, being powerless, full of conflict, dependent. All of these truths will lead you to find and grow your independent self, which you will do by relying on others and on your higher power. You'll still be a bundle of contradictions, and that's all just fine. These opposites within you may be troubling, but they're normal, understandable, and you'll have learned to live with all and none and plenty in the middle.

This new "selfishness," this new respect for yourself, will allow you to be a good person, a good wife or partner, a good mother, a good friend and colleague. You will be a better person in every respect as you refuse to give up yourself in bondage to another. You will also refuse to give up yourself to fix your pain, to squelch your needs and wishes. You will be able to say yes and to say no, and you will definitely be able to compromise. Having a self won't mean you have to have it all. Having a self will mean you have a choice. It will mean you must choose, all the time. When you choose, you will open yourself to claim and accept responsibility for your choice. You will open yourself to feel the good in what you have chosen and the loss for what you have left behind. You will open yourself to feel the guilt that you can't be all for everyone, and you may even feel guilt because you have survived. You didn't die. You didn't lose. You will have claimed the right to live by being sober.

Geri takes us home:

How do I say thank you? How do I ever express the gratitude for what I've been given? How do I explain the life I live now, and how do I tell anyone how I got here? I could have died. I should have died. And I did die inside. I never could have envisioned what I could be, what my life could be like, and how deeply secure and grateful I could feel. I was full of anger, full of hate, and out to fight my way through life. And then it was over. I couldn't do it anymore. I got the chance for recovery. I grabbed it and have been holding on ever since. I know that every single day I have the choice to stay sober. I have the choice to hold on to the healthy me I've grown through my sobriety. Or I can give me away. Anytime. It's a great freedom and a great responsibility. I accept.

Epilogue

I accept. Just like Geri. In that long ago moment when I knew that I had no choice except to drink, I got a choice—my first great gift of recovery. I have been stepping up to make that choice every day for more than thirty-two years. I have said yes to abstinence and no to drinking, day after day, year after year, always one step at a time.

Early on, I felt safely held and carried forward before I could know what was happening, or where I was going. I have been blessed to stay on this path even when I didn't understand. I was given a deep trust that I didn't have and couldn't muster for myself.

And so, I got all the gifts that Geri and Carole and Patti and Tenaya and all the other women in this book received. Most of all, I got the great gift of myself by staying on the road and in the process.

The big picture of my life as a sober woman is a story of slow, steady, positive change, punctuated by radical transformations, moments of new insight and new truths that would propel me into a completely different internal space and a new sense of myself. For me, thirty-two years of growth have been a combination of slow and steady, sharp and radical. From that point of starting over, on March 19, 1971, I have been slowly but surely coming into my self, and coming to live with others, above the ground.

Initially, in new sobriety, I lived in a surreal state. I couldn't see anything clearly except the stark reality of my own drinking, that moment, now branded on my soul, that I knew I had no choice. That I had had to do this. I had had to go through these rhythmic motions, day after day. Drink, drunk, do it all again.

I stayed sober day after day in a similar rhythmic way. Clarity came slowly. For years in recovery, I lived in an internal border zone of two worlds: the pure, absolute certainty of my alcoholism and my sober self, and the automatic, knee-jerk pull back to my old self and my old life, the underground, boozy swamp.

I carry the memory of my past, and sometimes I can feel the realities of my childhood and my own drinking life as if they were occurring in present time. Yet I am not pulled back, down, or under by remembering, as happened early on. Nostalgia no longer threatens. I feel the strength of my second self, the recovering self I've worked hard to grow over all these years. Now my dream state occurs mostly during sleep.

I got to grow a new me, a new self. I got to learn from scratch about myself and relationships that would not be formed by a mutual craving for alcohol and a love born and bred in a drunken haze. I got to work my way out of the alcoholic fog of my childhood life and that same world I repeated as a young adult.

Over the years, as I felt safe and secure in recovery, I could see more, and I could feel more. I could tolerate the awkwardness of learning how to walk and talk, of learning who I am through the lens and the language of recovery. I still had those raw impulses of drinking, but I gave them new expression in the rhythmic, repetitive actions of recovery. And they grew quieter, softer. Rat, tat, tat, like a drum roll, I followed this new way.

From a language of impulse to a language of recovery, I got new words that labeled reality and new feelings to match. I remembered, and I told the true story of my life as I got my feet on solid ground. Restraint, reflection, quietness, safety. The rat, tat, tat was slow and steady, and growth accumulated like inch marks crawling up the wall by the kitchen door. And then there were the giant leaps of transformation that have punctuated my growth over all these years. Like this one. With about a year of sobriety, I was feeling trapped in that border zone, stuck between two worlds and unable to see or know my way out. I stayed sober but felt a thick haze and a thick tongue. Why couldn't I move? Why couldn't I figure this out?

Then I had a dramatic insight. As a young teen, I played tennis, a sport I loved. But tennis gave way to adolescent partying, and I became a "former athlete" at a young age. When I stopped drinking, I decided to take up tennis again. I practiced by myself on a backboard, enjoying the rhythm of the thumping ball and my fairly consistent returns. One day in this meditative practice, I realized that I ran around my backhand a lot. Then I noticed that I didn't swing the way I had been taught. Over the course of several months at the backboard, I determined that I played "well enough." I could get the ball back and hit reasonably good shots. I felt okay about accepting my quirks of form and my decision to settle for "getting by."

Then it hit me, another of those blessed moments. As if I were once again standing at the kitchen sink with the glass in my hand, I knew I had a choice. I could accept my poor form and I could get by. Or I could start over and learn the correct form. I knew it would be hard to do and I knew it would take a lot of time and effort. And I knew I would play much worse as I was correcting my form and changing everything about the way I played. Could I tolerate all of this work, and could I tolerate bumbling and fumbling and playing poorly for however long it would take?

I decided in that moment to correct my form, and I have been working on my "corrected form" ever since. I do play a better game of tennis now, but I can go back to sloppy ways in a minute. Those old "quirks" are still there, but they're not all of me anymore.

In that moment I think I understood what recovery is about. I understood that I could stay stuck and "get by," but I also chose not to. Getting by was not what I wanted anymore.

This experience of transformation is, of course, a metaphor. I've had many more of these wondrous moments, times when I could see myself and face myself clearly and know the "truth" in that split second. I've also had times where "getting by" was a right choice, where I could accept my limits and know that settling for less was a healthy choice. That acceptance did not mean that I was giving up or betraying myself.

Slow and steady growth has been the underlying thread, the step-by-step forward path. When I had been sober for twelve years and my present, real life was solid and good, I started to cry one day as I was describing my childhood and my days of drinking. I cried, it seems, for the next twelve years—slow and steady—whenever I spoke about my past. I had a lot to cry about, and now it was safe enough to let it out. I would not make that border crossing back into active drinking or the loss of myself. These were now tears of sorrow, regret, loss, relief, and deep gratitude.

This was a long haul, and there were times I thought that this couldn't be recovery. Yet I knew I had done the work of growing a new me so I could feel the pain. Only then could I feel the joys of my life and live in the now.

That is what happened. One day the crying of my past stopped and I stepped above the ground to see an expansive world and to feel the security of a grown-up me. I could feel my limits, my dependence, my great freedom, and my deep responsibility, while trusting in the greater good.

Years before, a dream had opened the door.

There I was, sitting calmly, sorrowfully, amid the bones. Just skeletal remains. I was going nowhere. In this dream, I was stationed underground, in the grave, a sentry and a partner. This was my company, my life, my mission—to watch over the bones.

And then slowly, but quite purposefully, I got up. I walked away and climbed out of the grave, into the sun and the wide expanse of the world that was there waiting for me. I turned one last time to say good-bye. The vigil of the bones was over.

I am still going slow and steady, with sudden flashes of life-changing insight. This is my life, and I am grateful.

Stephanie Brown
November 2003

The Twelve Steps of Alcoholics Anonymous*

1. We admitted we were powerless over alcohol—that our lives had become unmanageable.
2. Came to believe that a Power greater than ourselves could restore us to sanity.
3. Made a decision to turn our will and our lives over to the care of God *as we understood Him.*
4. Made a searching and fearless moral inventory of ourselves.
5. Admitted to God, to ourselves, and to another human being the exact nature of our wrongs.
6. Were entirely ready to have God remove all these defects of character.
7. Humbly asked Him to remove our shortcomings.
8. Made a list of all persons we had harmed, and became willing to make amends to them all.
9. Made direct amends to such people wherever possible, except when to do so would injure them or others.
10. Continued to take personal inventory and when we were wrong promptly admitted it.
11. Sought through prayer and meditation to improve our conscious contact with God *as we understood Him,* praying only for knowledge of His will for us and the power to carry that out.
12. Having had a spiritual awakening as the result of these steps, we tried to carry this message to alcoholics, and to practice these principles in all our affairs.

*From *Alcoholics Anonymous,* 4th ed., published by AA World Services, Inc., New York, N.Y., 59–60.

The Twelve Traditions of Alcoholics Anonymous*

1. Our common welfare should come first; personal recovery depends upon A.A. unity.
2. For our group purpose there is but one ultimate authority—a loving God as He may express Himself in our group conscience. Our leaders are but trusted servants; they do not govern.
3. The only requirement for A.A. membership is a desire to stop drinking.
4. Each group should be autonomous except in matters affecting other groups or A.A. as a whole.
5. Each group has but one primary purpose—to carry its message to the alcoholic who still suffers.
6. An A.A. group ought never endorse, finance, or lend the A.A. name to any related facility or outside enterprise, lest problems of money, property, and prestige divert us from our primary purpose.
7. Every A.A. group ought to be fully self-supporting, declining outside contributions.
8. Alcoholics Anonymous should remain forever nonprofessional, but our service centers may employ special workers.
9. A.A., as such, ought never be organized; but we may create service boards or committees directly responsible to those they serve.
10. Alcoholics Anonymous has no opinion on outside issues; hence our A.A. name ought never be drawn into public controversy.
11. Our public relations policy is based on attraction rather than promotion; we need always maintain personal anonymity at the level of press, radio, and films.
12. Anonymity is the spiritual foundation of all our traditions, ever reminding us to place principles before personalities.

*From *Twelve Steps and Twelve Traditions*, published by AA World Services, Inc., New York, N.Y., 129–187.

About the Author

Stephanie Brown, Ph.D., is a pioneering researcher, clinician, author, teacher, and consultant in the addiction field. A psychologist, she is the director of the Addictions Institute, Menlo Park, California, where she has a private practice. She is a research associate at the Mental Research Institute in Palo Alto, where she codirects the Family Recovery Research Project. Dr. Brown is the author of eight books. She most recently coedited *The Handbook of Addiction Treatment for Women: Theory and Practice*.

Hazelden Foundation, a national nonprofit organization founded in 1949, helps people reclaim their lives from the disease of addiction. Built on decades of knowledge and experience, Hazelden's comprehensive approach to addiction addresses the full range of individual, family, and professional needs, including addiction treatment and continuing care services for youth and adults, publishing, research, higher learning, public education, and advocacy.

A life of recovery is lived "one day at a time." Hazelden publications, both educational and inspirational, support and strengthen lifelong recovery. In 1954, Hazelden published *Twenty-Four Hours a Day,* the first daily meditation book for recovering alcoholics, and Hazelden continues to publish works to inspire and guide individuals in treatment and recovery, and their loved ones. Professionals who work to prevent and treat addiction also turn to Hazelden for evidence-based curricula, informational materials, and videos for use in schools, treatment programs, and correctional programs.

Through published works, Hazelden extends the reach of hope, encouragement, help, and support to individuals, families, and communities affected by addiction and related issues.

For questions about Hazelden publications, please call **800-328-9000** or visit us online at **hazelden.org/bookstore.**